A Practical Guide to

Documentation in Behavioral Health Care

Third Edition

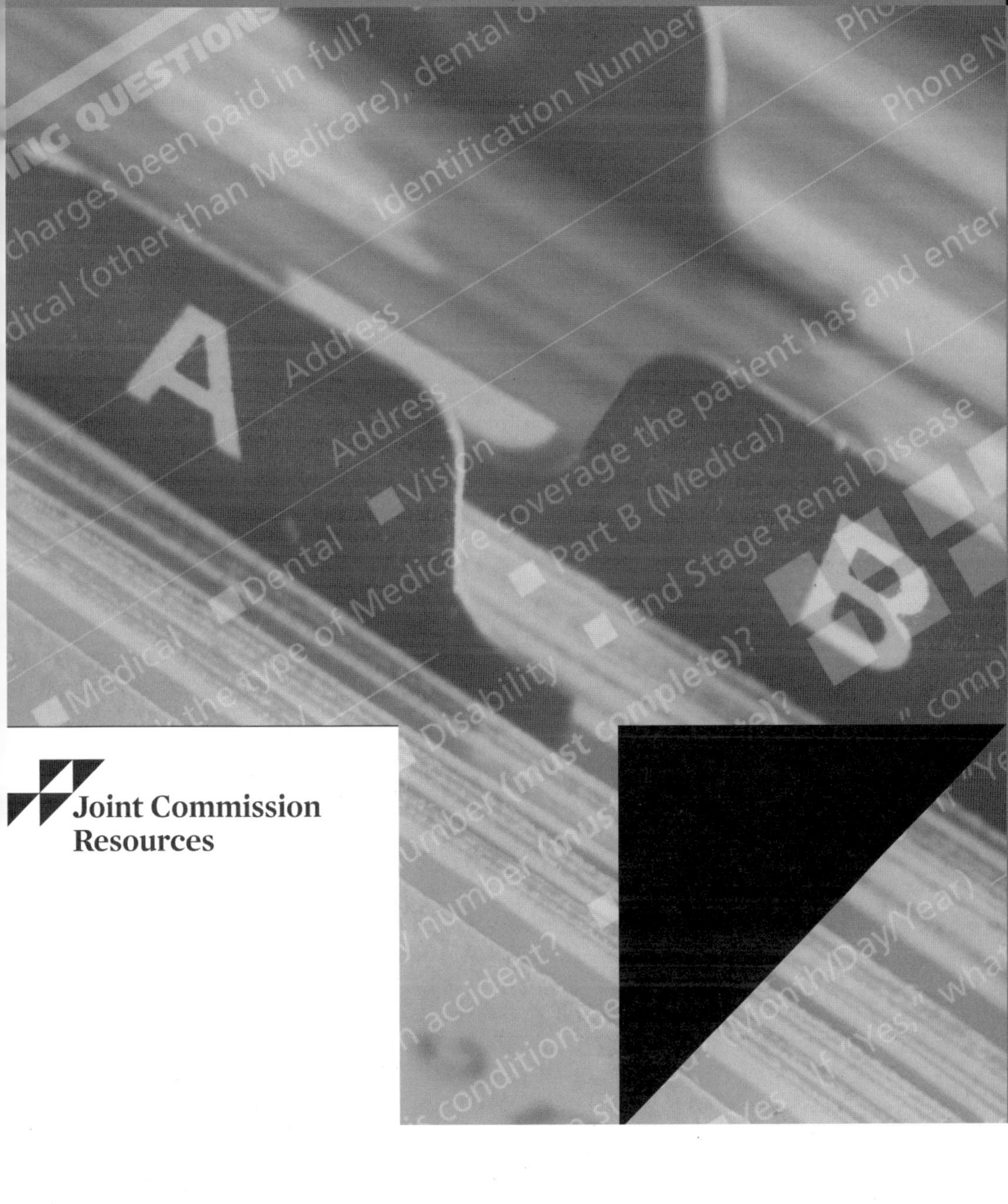

Joint Commission Resources

Senior Editor: Audrie Bretl
Senior Project Manager: Cheryl Firestone
Manager, Publications: Paul Reis
Associate Director, Production: Johanna Harris
Associate Director, Editorial Development: Diane Bell
Executive Director: Catherine Chopp Hinckley, Ph.D.
Vice President, Learning: Charles Macfarlane, F.A.C.H.E.
Joint Commission/JCR Reviewers: Mary Cesare-Murphy, Peggy Lavin, Merlin Wessels, Paul Reis

Joint Commission Resources Mission

The mission of Joint Commission Resources is to continuously improve the safety and quality of care in the United States and in the international community through the provision of education and consultation services and international accreditation.

Joint Commission Resources educational programs and publications support, but are separate from, the accreditation activities of The Joint Commission. Attendees at Joint Commission Resources educational programs and purchasers of Joint Commission Resources publications receive no special consideration or treatment in, or confidential information about, the accreditation process.

The inclusion of an organization name, product, or service in a Joint Commission publication should not be construed as an endorsement of such organization, product, or service, nor is failure to include an organization name, product, or service to be construed as disapproval.

This publication is designed to provide accurate and authoritative information in regard to the subject matter covered. Every attempt has been made to ensure accuracy at the time of publication; however, please note that laws, regulations, and standards are subject to change. Please also note that some of the examples in this publication are specific to the laws and regulations of the locality of the facility. The information and examples in this publication are provided with the understanding that the publisher is not engaged in providing medical, legal, or other professional advice. If any such assistance is desired, the services of a competent professional person should be sought.

Printed in the U.S.A. 5 4 3 2 1

Requests for permission to make copies of any part of this work should be mailed to
Permissions Editor
Department of Publications
Joint Commission Resources
One Renaissance Boulevard
Oakbrook Terrace, Illinois 60181
permissions@jcrinc.com

ISBN: 978-1-59940-186-7
Library of Congress Control Number: 2007941266

For more information about Joint Commission Resources, please visit http://www.jcrinc.com.

Contents

Introduction

In its introduction to the "Management of Information" chapter in the *Comprehensive Accreditation Manual for Behavioral Health Care,* The Joint Commission states that an organization's "provision of care, treatment, and services is a complex endeavor that is highly dependent on information." While information can manifest itself in verbal, observed, and textual ways, in the case of documentation, that information comprises a permanent record of a client's experience as he or she navigates the behavioral health care organization.

Documentation is the means by which the knowledge and information about the organization's clients is prepared and stored. Without documentation, the organization might still provide care, treatment, and services, but the continuity and effectiveness of that care could be severely impaired. Staff may end up providing conflicting or repetitive care steps to clients, crucial initial assessment information gleaned from the client could be lost, reimbursement channels could be diminished, and any sense of progress could appear inconsistent or lacking.

A behavioral health care organization can and does use documentation for a number of reasons, including, but not limited to, the following:

- Initial assessments and screenings
- Reassessments
- Continuity of care
- Plan of care
- Discharge planning
- Interdisciplinary team collaboration
- Intraorganization communication
- Reimbursement and coding
- Record review and referral processes
- Staff education and mentoring
- Equipment and/or resource management
- Holding both the client and clinician responsible in the treatment process
- Protecting the organization from malpractice

In addition, behavioral health care organizations are required to maintain documentation to comply with specific regulatory bodies, such as state and/or authorities like the Centers for Medicare & Medicaid Services, and accrediting bodies, such as the Joint Commission. Although the Joint Commission does not delineate a specific style or approach to documentation, it does lay out a series of expectations and requirements in its standards relating to documentation.

The process of effective care, treatment, and services should be the primary driver behind an organization's documentation design. Documentation should exist to support the delivery of high-quality care to clients. To that end, organizations should work to ensure that both processes support each other and work to maximize the efforts of the organization. When used from this standpoint, documentation can be seen as an aid to the organization's overall mission and goals.

How a behavioral health care organization prepares, collects, and uses its documentation can have an impact on how well that organization functions. This presents an imperative to ensure that an organization's documentation is consistent, precise, and well prepared. This imperative must cover all types of documentation that an organization might prepare, including the following:

- Initial assessments
- Planning of care
- Progress notes
- Discharge planning
- Multidisciplinary team meeting notes

A Practical Guide to Documentation in Behavioral Health Care, Third Edition, was developed to help providers document care events more efficiently and effectively. It encourages more practical and useful documentation for providers, clients, and those who financially support client care. This publication encourages behavioral health care professionals to accept the premise that skillful documentation improves care, treatment, and services and can be considered as important as competence when providing care. It does not favor a particular care orientation, nor does it encourage the use of one philosophical approach over another. In addition, this publication seeks to present the important principles and concepts that guide effective documentation. As a result, while not all forms or examples presented in this book are applicable to all types of behavioral health care organizations, the concepts and principles should resonate in all types of settings.

COMMUNICATION: THE DRIVER OF DOCUMENTATION

The clinical/case record is intended to communicate significant information in a language that is understandable to all who have access to the file. It is essential, therefore, that the material be written simply and clearly. It is hoped that this publication will help with that task.

In addition to the need for effective communication (and documentation) for the sake of effective client care, client safety must also be considered. Based on sentinel event data received at the Joint Commission, the root cause analyses of the majority of reported sentinel events found that breakdowns in communication were the leading cause of those errors.[1] The need for effective and well-planned communication is driven not only by a desire for providing high-quality care, treatment, and services, but also to ensure that it is as safe as possible.

PROVIDERS' VERBAL STYLE VERSUS WRITTEN STYLE

Although providers may have differing opinions about the cause of a client's behavior, there is rarely any dissent about the characteristics of the behavior itself. Unfortunately, the clarity and specificity of the oral language is not often carried over to the written clinical/case record of the client. Assessment statements, the needs of the client, care goals, and care objectives are written in language very different from that used during everyday discussions. Often, global terms are used to document the behavior. Sometimes only a diagnosis is recorded. In other instances, the language or terminology of a particular discipline is used, and this language may be unclear to professionals from other disciplines. Most important, the lack of specificity or the use of jargon may confuse the client, with whom the plan of care, goals, and objectives are shared. This book encourages the use of "plain" or "clear" English rather than global or all-encompassing terminology in documentation. Using practical and simple language will help those involved in documentation to accomplish the following:

- Communicate to the client, other professionals, and payers what, where, when, how, and why care, treatment, or service events occur
- Establish a road map for progress

- Monitor progress
- Establish a means for measuring organization and provider performance for the purpose of improvement
- Establish a database for management information systems and research
- Devote less time to paperwork and more to direct care of the client

One of the great benefits of practical language is that it simplifies not only the documentation but also the perceptual framework of providing care. In the current behavioral health care environment, with its emphasis on cost reduction, providers everywhere are constrained to focus more on neutralizing a target behavior than attaining an enhanced quality of life for the client. From the time of their first interaction with the client, providers are pressured to identify why the individual needs care, what care will most rapidly modify the behavior or will most effectively produce behavioral change, and how long it will take. The simpler the language used to clarify care issues, the more quickly providers can facilitate care, treatment, or services.

THE IMPERATIVE FOR PRECISE DOCUMENTATION

As a key method of communication in a behavioral health care organization, the more precise, comprehensive, and clear the documentation is, the less chance there will be for confusion, incorrect treatment, or errors in treatment, all of which can lead to adverse outcomes.

In recent years, health care effectiveness and efficiency—particularly in behavioral health care—have become volatile topics within the national dialogue on health issues. One consequence of the economic constraints imposed on behavioral health care expenditures of late is that those who provide care are being required to demonstrate to their clients, to payers, and to themselves that their care, treatment, or service outcomes are achieved prudently, ethically, and with efficacy. To do this, there must be a source of solid information that clearly delineates what changes occurred (for example, outcomes) as the result of the investment of resources, both human and fiscal. The data source must distinctly describe the client; describe what was provided during care, treatment, or service; and describe the client either upon completion of such care, treatment, or service or upon transfer.

The most logical place to find such concrete evidence should be the clinical/case record. That is the storage site for the salient information about the behavior of the client before care; what care, treatment, or service was delivered to improve the behaviors; how a response to that care has been progressing; and what the behaviors were. If the record of the client lacks specificity, outcome data will lack specificity, and it will be impossible to substantiate the effectiveness and efficacy of care, treatment, or service.

In the not-too-distant past, concerns about the quality of the clinical/case record were generally confined to the providers. It was not that administrative staff were disinterested in the clinical/case record of the client, but in most instances the quality of documentation indirectly affected administrative and managerial functions or the survival of the organization. It was also the case that clinical/case records customarily received the most attention shortly before the scheduled visit of licensing or accrediting bodies.

This situation has changed drastically. Today, the quality and content of the clinical/case record may well determine whether care, treatment, or service is deemed appropriate and whether that level of care, treatment, or service is justified and reimbursable. The determination of whether reimbursement will occur at all may be based solely on what is written—and in some instances, what is not written—in the clinical/case record. The quality of documentation may ultimately determine whether an organization can survive financially.

The quality and content of the clinical/case record may also play a role in how well the client's treatment plan is carried out. Ambiguities, missing documentation, or poorly written records can adversely impact how well an organization works together to care for the client. Also, if certain steps in the documentation process, such as the preparation of progress notes or the use of multidisciplinary notes or planning meetings are missing or inadequate, the quality of how well care, treatment, and services progresses could be compromised. In the worst-case scenario, an error could take place that could actually compromise the health and well-being of the client.

EXTERNAL PRESSURES FOR QUALITY DOCUMENTATION

Consumer demands for accountability in behavioral health care have increased over the past several years, and it is unlikely that they will diminish. Providers should be using systems that help to generate great amounts of objective data. Unfortunately, insufficient data are available to help consumers make decisions, particularly from behavioral health care providers. To establish reliable databases that reflect their efforts, providers should improve their ability to record care processes and results (that is, outcomes). Sophisticated management information systems and computerized clinical/case records are helpful tools, but they are only as reliable as the information fed into them. The clinical/case record must be capable of serving as the primary database for the client. The record should clearly identify the following:

- The condition (that is, behaviors) of the client
- Presenting problems or needs (that is, behaviors) that will be addressed during care, those that will be referred to other providers, and those that will be deferred to another time
- Why the care, treatment, or service is necessary; the setting is appropriate; and alternative interventions are not considered appropriate
- The changes anticipated for the client (that is, goals and objectives) and their anticipated achievement time frames (that is, target dates)
- The care, treatment, or service provided to modify or eliminate the behaviors (for example, interventions) or meet the needs of the clients and the required frequency of services
- The condition (outcome) of the client after care, treatment, or service
- The plan to address the individual's ongoing needs (that is, transfer, discharge, or aftercare plan)

The record should contain additional critical material. It should also reveal the following:

- The benefit received in return for the outlay of resources (that is, cost-effectiveness)
- Justification for the outlay of resources (that is, cost-efficiency)

These are not new issues for behavioral health care professionals. Most providers have been generating data, and others have earnestly improved their management information systems in response to customer pressures. The external pressure for the questions to be answered objectively and supported by data continues.

Many providers need to enhance their perceptions about the need for—and value of—documentation if valid outcome data are to be generated. To evaluate outcomes, the documented language must be precise and measurable. Outcomes must be described in observable terms. As the written language is freed of ambiguity, the outcomes, cost-efficiency, and cost-effectiveness of care, treatment, and services can be more readily calculated. As the allocation of precious and dwindling resources becomes increasingly based on demonstrable need, superior documentation will become a routine expectation. Organizations will increasingly require every provider to competently record every clinical/case record entry. Quality documentation should not be correlated with a visit from a licensing body or accrediting organization; it should be expected of every provider, every day, and at every level of care.

With growing frequency, external reviewers look to documentation to justify the delivery of care and reimbursement because there is no richer source of justification. There is almost always some level of review before beginning care, treatment, or service at all levels. Precertification review is a virtual certainty for almost all levels of care, treatment, and service. Other formal record reviews are conducted concurrently with care, treatment, and service, or retrospectively. Whether an organization receives payment for the care it renders has increasingly become linked to the quality of care, treatment, and service documentation. Even the most skilled providers will be unable to render care if their income is eliminated because of reimbursement denials tied to inadequate documentation.

The external forces that are pressuring providers to convincingly support the need for care, treatment, and services cannot be minimized. The most powerful argument for quality clinical/case recording is very simply stated: Quality documentation facilitates quality care.

ADVOCACY ON BEHALF OF CLIENTS

The ability to efficiently and effectively record the needs, strengths, and progress of the client unburdens providers and allows them to devote more time to the client. The ability to clearly communicate the nature of the target behaviors of the client and the measures that can be taken to bring them under control should be very comforting to the client, as it helps him or her understand that improvement is not only achievable, but likely. The more similar the provider's language to that of the client, the more likely the client will participate in the plan of care.

Quality documentation enables organizations to evaluate and improve processes and outcomes by relying on the clinical/case record as a data resource. The results of evaluation may precipitate performance improvement enterprises or staff development activities, resulting in better care for those being served.

PUBLICATION OVERVIEW

A Practical Guide to Documentation in Behavioral Health Care, Third Edition, is an updated edition of the widely used and appreciated publication that shares tips and strategies on how to effectively prepare, use, and analyze documentation. With updated content and added features, this publication is divided into the following three sections:

- *Section 1: The Process and Structure of Care* discusses care as a continuous process that consists of data collection, data assessment, action planning, and action implementation. It also explores issues relating to the need for good documentation, the use of electronic records, coding and reimbursement, and confidentiality, privacy, and security issues relating to documentation.
- *Section 2: The Process and Structure of Screening/Assessment* discusses screening and assessment, including such components as physical, psychosocial, nutritional, spiritual, and vocational. Also addressed are analysis of the significant data gathered from physical and

psychosocial screenings/assessments of the client into a single evaluation, problems/needs lists, and the importance of precise language.

- *Section 3: The Process and Structure of Planning of Care* discusses aspects of planning care; progress notes; plan reviews; continuing care, treatment, or service plans; practice guidelines where available, and documentation competence. In addition, this section looks at regulatory and accreditation requirements in relation to documentation and performance improvement and documentation.

Examples of good documentation skills are included and analyzed in all three sections of the book. An Appendix, consisting of a collection of sample forms that can be adapted to suit your organization, is also included on the CD at the back of the book. It is important to note that the examples are just that—examples. The examples and tools provided are not the only possible way to meet the intent of the standards in every type of behavioral health care organization that the Joint Commission accredits. The reader is urged to share the examples with the appropriate staff. However, the examples need to be reviewed, approved, or modified as necessary by the organizations' service leaders if implemented for their own use. The forms mentioned throughout the publication are included on an accompanying CD-ROM for your use and easy reference.

New in the Third Edition

This updated edition includes the following:

- Additional forms and examples in the Appendix on the included CD-ROM, representing a broad spectrum of behavioral health care organizations
- New material and discussion on coding and reimbursement, privacy and security in documentation, client safety and documentation, and accreditation-related requirements
- Enhanced and/or newly added content on the principles of good and precise documentation, electronic records, performance improvement, and documentation in specific situations for specific types of health care settings
- New case examples from organizations on how they are using documentation to enhance their ongoing delivery of care, treatment, and services

The third edition of *A Practical Guide to Documentation* is intended for caregivers and leaders wanting to improve their documentation skills. It is hoped that after reading this material, providers will recognize that weak documentation is a waste of valuable time and does nothing to improve care, treatment, or service. Weak documentation can also diminish the quality of care by compelling skilled providers to devote inordinate time and energy trying to either clarify or understand what has been written (or not written) and that detracts from the valuable time available to care for the clients. It takes unnecessary time—and possibly more—to deal with the consequences of poorly written documentation.

About the Terms Used in This Publication

Throughout the spectrum of what has been referred to as behavioral health care services, certain terms referring to those receiving care, treatment, and services and those who are providing that care can and do differ. For the sake of simplicity and clarity, this publication will refer to those who provide care in such settings as acute care, residential/group homes, transitional/supervised/ supportive living, therapeutic foster care, foster care, corrections, forensics, day programs, family preservation/wraparound, case management, in-home, outpatient, vocational rehabilitation, shelters, online, outdoor, and opioid treatment programs, simply as *behavioral health care organizations*. The exception to that will be when the publication is describing a specific type of program or setting. In addition, while the field of behavioral health care may use terms such as *youth, child, patient,* or *client* to describe those individuals who receive care, treatment, and services from certain types of behavioral health care organizations, this publication will use the term *client* unless specifically describing an individual receiving care at a specific kind of behavioral health care organization or when quoting specific material or referring to forms from specific types of health care organizations.

ACKNOWLEDGEMENTS

The development of a publication depends on the input and expertise of many individuals and perspectives. Joint Commission Resources (JCR) wishes to thank the many organizations and individuals who provided their expert insight and guidance into the development of this book in all its editions either as content experts, reviewers, or profiled organizations. Particular thanks go to those organizations and individuals who granted their permission for JCR to use the material and many forms and examples that enhance the quality of this work and help it achieve its potential. Thanks also to the reviewers of this publication for ensuring accuracy and completeness, Hillel Bodek for his expertise and resources, and to Ladan Cockshut for her writing talents.

REFERENCE

1. Joint Commission: *Sentinel Event.* 2007. http://www.jointcommission.org/sentinelevents (accessed Oct. 5, 2007).

Section 1

THE PROCESS AND STRUCTURE OF CARE

Care, treatment, and services are processes of interrelated functions. These processes can also be perceived as an integrated system of processes and outcomes. It can best be conceptualized, however, as a system composed of four basic elements: data collection, data assessment, action planning, and action implementation (*see* Figure 1-1, page 2).

Care, treatment, and services are not a sequence of independent events. To ensure that the four elements identified in Figure 1-1 are being conducted effectively, one uses important decision points (or checkpoints) during the care process that are sometimes incorrectly considered events. Staff may refer to them as if they were discrete and isolated activities. For example, staff may report that they are scheduled to "attend planning of care" or meeting to "do an assessment." Referring to a process in this manner can establish the impression that it is a stand-alone event. In reality, it is a formalized checkpoint within processes that never cease. Examples of such events include the following:

- Intake process
- Screening for needed assessing
- Biopsychosocial assessment(s)
- Analysis and integration of significant care data into one evaluation (or clinical formulation)
- Plan of care
- Continuing plan of care

Each event actually constitutes only a short pause in the continuous chain of processes that have preceded it and will follow it. Sometimes structured checkpoints are thought of as events because they generally occur according to expectations established at the time of planning of care. Or, they are guided by organization policies and procedures. The emergence of managed care has reduced some of the inflexibility related to the processes. Frequent—sometimes daily—reviews of the condition of the client are customarily necessary to justify continued care, treatment, or service.

Systems are designed and planned. They possess structure and are controlled by guiding principles. They are characterized by flexibility. Systems are developed to achieve specific, predetermined outcomes. Because of their flexibility, they can be tailored to different styles of use and varied types of users.

Large systems are generally composed of subsystems defined by the same characteristics. Subsystems may be further broken down. For example, at one time, behavioral health care providers tended to confine their energies to delivering only one level of care, treatment, or service: the system of residential care. The system was relatively uncomplicated. Today, increasing numbers of providers are expanding the levels of care they offer. Organizations that once provided only residential services have expanded to provide a broader and improved continuum of care. A single care system is now composed of subsystems, such as crisis stabilization, residential, day treatment, outpatient, opioid

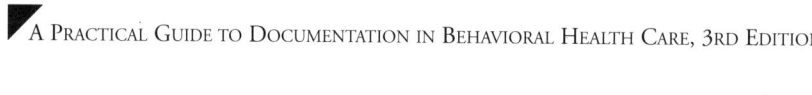
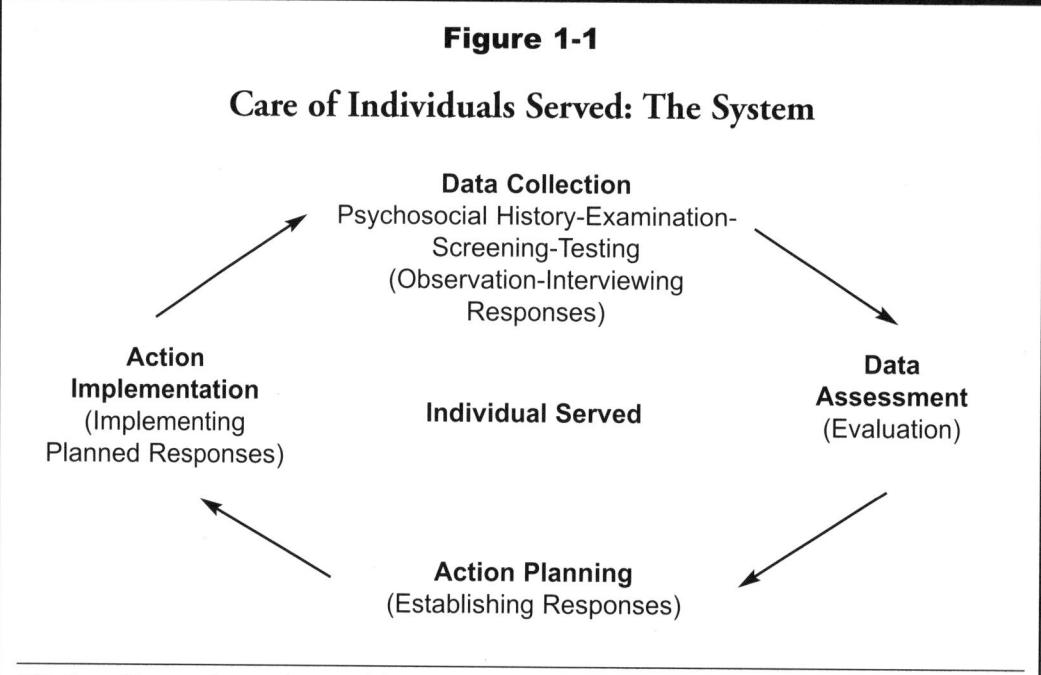

Figure 1-1

Care of Individuals Served: The System

Data Collection
Psychosocial History-Examination-
Screening-Testing
(Observation-Interviewing
Responses)

**Action
Implementation**
(Implementing
Planned Responses)

Individual Served

**Data
Assessment**
(Evaluation)

Action Planning
(Establishing Responses)

This figure illustrates the core elements of the care assessment system for individuals served.

Source: Joint Commission Resources: *A Practical Guide to Documentation in Behavioral Health Care,* 2nd ed. Oakbrook Terrace, IL: The Joint Commission, 2002.

treatment programs, and home-based services, such as wraparound, foster care, parenting classes, adoption, and behavioral health promotion.

The care process itself is also composed of interlinking processes. The elements identified in Figure 1-1, above, are examples of subsystems within the larger system of care.

The quality of any multilevel system is a function of the quality of the subsystems; any change in the quality of a subsystem affects the quality of each of the other subsystems as well as the quality of the larger system of care.

THE BASIC ELEMENTS OF CARE, TREATMENT, AND SERVICES

The core process of care, treatment, and services generally involves the continuous interaction of specific components in the same sequence; however, there are refinements, and some elements may be revisited repeatedly, as warranted. An abbreviated description of the steps follows. Each step is discussed in greater depth in subsequent sections.

Data Collection

Data are collected about the history of the client, current behaviors, and past and existing physical, emotional, and behavioral functioning. In most instances, the data are collected directly by the providers within a single site and level of care. When specialty testing or examinations are required, they are usually obtained from external providers who have been deemed competent by the organization's clinical/service and administrative leadership. Data are gathered as quickly as possible so that the other activities in the process of care can be initiated without delay. The process of gathering initial information marks the beginning of care and constitutes the first engagement of the client in the care process. It may be initiated on site with a member of the care team or instituted by an intake staff person by telephone.

Screening

Screening is a brief process to identify life domains that need further assessment to guide care, treatment, and services. During the transition from data collection to data assessment, it may be appropriate to discuss screening to avoid confusion. In the behavioral health care field, there are a few types of screening that differ in approach:

Clerical: A screening clerk or secretary may gather some initial data on the client. This interview may be done face-to-face or over the telephone. The data collected are usually restricted to identification-type data, but they may also include some clinical data, usually limited to the source of and reason for referral. This data collection does not flow into data assessment, with perhaps one exception. It may be that the program has defined the population that will be admitted and treated as being limited to adults age 18–64. As a result, a 16-year-old student presented for admission may be inappropriate for admission due to his or her age. In this and similar cases, data collection and assessment may lead to a decision on admission and treatment despite an age discrepancy.

Data collection: A person may come into the program and provide required data by completing assessment forms, questionnaires, tests, and other evaluations. These may also include information such as legal processes and court referrals. In this type of screening, data collection does not flow into data assessment. The actual assessment of the data and the admission/treatment decision will take place at a later time or at a different location.

Meeting: A client meets with a clinical professional, and data are collected and assessed to determine the appropriateness of admission and treatment. During this process, the assessment of the data is the most comprehensive. The assessment is based on the data, the presentation of information such as eye contact, tone and level of voice, and demeanor. The clinical staff person uses all aspects of data in the assessment process.

Data Assessment

After the psychosocial and physical data have been gathered, they are assessed (that is, evaluated). It is important to note that although the formal assessment occurs shortly after the psychosocial and physical[1] assessments are completed, the data are evaluated at the same time. The difference between collecting data and evaluating it is also important to note. *Assessment* means collecting data, thoroughly evaluating it, and then drawing conclusions about its impact on the client. This is much more extensive than merely gathering (or collecting) the data to be evaluated.

Providers strive to understand the individual's behavior and the factors causing it, but they do not judge the individual's moral fiber. Furthermore, clinical/service assessments focus on how behavior creates difficulty or is a source of strength for the client rather than how it causes difficulty for those gathering the information or others. The professional assessment focuses on the client.

At the more intense levels of care (such as crisis stabilization units in community mental health centers, residential, and day treatment), the client is usually evaluated by a variety of professionals with expertise in one of the physical, psychological, or social dimensions. For example, nurses and physicians apply their special knowledge and skills to evaluate the physical dimension. Psychologists, psychiatrists, clinical social workers, and mental health counselors focus on the psychological dimension, whereas social workers, counselors, rehabilitation specialists, and others possessing specialized expertise assess the social dimension.

Action Planning

Action planning is initiated using a number of subsets of information from the data collection and assessment, including the following:

1. The data prepared by the client or by both the client and clinical staff (such as forms, histories, and questionnaires)

2. The data obtained by the clinical staff from assessment of the data. For example, if the individual is seeking treatment for alcohol or drug abuse, data concerning "history and patterns of alcohol or drug use" will allow the clinical staff to determine where the individual is within the "cycle of dependence." This may provide more data for action planning.

3. The actual absence of data can also be an important part of action planning. Securing these missing data would be a factor in action planning. There are other functional areas (such as nutritional, vocational, and legal) in which knowledge may be limited, and further assessment may be indicated.

4. The clinical process of data collection may also provide information for action planning. In addiction programs, for example, it is fairly common to find that during the intake session, the individual denies any "history of physical or sexual abuse." The clinical staff will determine that this issue should be reviewed at a later time based on the facts that the individual "avoided eye contact and appeared uncomfortable" discussing the issue. In all programs, data collection and analysis should also indicate the role of the family of the client in the action plan.

5. The clinical assessment of priorities necessary to complete a clinical case formulation or diagnostic summary. This process uses the data gathered through the assessment (as outlined above) and the information and knowledge obtained through the education, training, and experience of the clinical staff.

Using the information in the analysis of significant data from all screenings/assessments, the provider or care team prioritizes the needs of the client and formulates a plan of action in a written plan of care. As additional data are retrieved and further assessments are completed, the new information is used to supplement the initial plan.

When an organization uses a multidisciplinary approach and the first formal planning of care session is convened, any existing plan that has been activated (such as an initial plan that may have been prepared by the intake clinician) should be reviewed.

Unachieved goals and objectives are evaluated. Those requiring continued attention are included with the plan that is being developed. The plan of care should be reviewed on a scheduled basis, as well as whenever any significant change in the condition of the client warrants possible revision of the plan. The client should be involved in developing his or her plan of care. Participation can be accomplished in a number of ways, but active participation is critical. In some instances, the client sits in on the plan of care session as an active participant. In other situations, the primary staff may review the plan with the client before the formal plan of care session or review it with the client after the proposed plan has been completed. Whatever the method, the client should be familiar with the goals and objectives and should understand why they were established, what they mean, and how they will be achieved. The Joint Commission standards specify that "Clients are involved in decisions about care, treatment, and services provided."

It is insufficient to simply have the client's signature on the plan of care without further involvement in the process. Active participation by the client is required and can be easily reflected by a descriptive progress note. When a multidisciplinary model is not used, the provider discusses the care plan with the client. Sidebar 1-1, below, illustrates an example of how to document a client's involvement in planning of care. It is also important to note that without the client's involvement in treatment planning, the focus of treatment may not be what the client is interested in, resulting in low motivation to change or the client dropping out of treatment.

Action Implementation

Providers should deliver the planned care activities (methods/interventions) identified in the plan and in accordance with the documented anticipated time frames. Occasionally, the client is given reading, writing, or other assignments to help bring about behavioral change. A monitoring mechanism should ensure that these assignments are completed because they are considered planned care activities (methods/interventions).

As a routine part of their responsibilities, providers should continuously evaluate the effectiveness of the care methods/interventions and determine whether the frequency, type, or intensity of service should be modified. The scope of the review is particularly important if the client does not appear to be responding. The review should always include a determination of whether the planned care activities were actually carried out as detailed in the written plan.

In the written guidelines or standards of licensing agencies, payers, and regulatory bodies, the process of care is often divided into subsystems of a larger system. Processes such as screenings/assessments, planning of care, and continuing plan of care are separate in many licensing and accrediting standards, which are often reviewed separately from one another (although The

---

Sidebar 1-1

Involvement of a Client in Planning of Care

Individual involvement in planning of care:
John actively participated in his planning of care by sharing his ideas on what he wanted from his care, as well as by providing feedback to staff on his goals and objectives. John has established a short-term objective and eventually would like to be employed.

Individual understanding of planning of care:
John has agreed that his plan of care captures first steps toward his goal of independent living.

Individual agreement with planning of care:
John agrees with all goals except the anger management goal. Mary Jones, John's counselor, will address this issue on an individual basis with him.

Joint Commission does not view these processes as isolated steps). An unintended outcome of such a process can be the erroneous impression that each is a singular event that has no relationship to the other steps in the care process. In reality, each is merely a checkpoint to track whether or not the care process is productive.

The administrative separation of the process of care into its individual parts is necessary and reasonable in order to effectively respond to the demands of managed care entities, third-party payers, and external review entities. Moreover, by conducting program evaluation at the defined points, vital organization functions such as performance improvement, quality control, risk management, information management, and usage review can be more efficiently accomplished. The decision points can also be used as terminals for evaluation activities such as peer review, supervision, performance appraisals (including competency assessments), and staff development.

Staff may reach the false conclusion that when the required steps (such as analysis of significant information about the client) have been completed, diminished attention to the quality of subsequent documentation is permissible. This may partially explain why many staff perceive assessment summaries, planning of care sessions, and discharge planning reviews as agonizing but necessary events rather than as important checkpoints within a continuous process of care.

THE COMPONENTS OF THE CARE PROCESS
Initial Contact Screening
Care is a seamless process that begins with the first contact and concludes with the last contact with the client. When a client makes the initial contact with a provider, sufficient preliminary data should be gathered to determine the appropriate provider, site, and level of care. Using the structure depicted in Figure 1-2 on page 7, sufficient data should be collected and evaluated to determine whether the level of care, treatment, or service is appropriate. If the evaluation reveals that the client is appropriate for care and that the required services are available and accessible, the next step in the process can be planned and implemented. The material gathered during the initial contact screening interview includes at least the following:

- Presenting conditions/needs that relate to the reason the individual is seeking or has been referred for care, treatment, or service
- Current strengths and preferences
- Level of acuity and duration of presenting needs/condition
- Basic demographics (such as age and sex)
- Funding source, if required

The evaluation of these data may reveal that a referral to a different provider is prudent. But assuming that the individual's condition meets the program's documented intake/admission criteria, the intake/admission assessment (data collection) session is convened, the data are assessed (evaluated), a plan of action is initiated, and intake/admission (action) is implemented.

Physical and Psychosocial Assessments
The individual's physical and psychosocial functioning is assessed to identify the strengths and needs of the client and to develop and activate the plan of care. In crisis stabilization units and residential settings, the assessment process is begun immediately upon admission to promptly identify whether any life-threatening conditions (risk to self or others) requiring immediate intervention exist. In less intense levels of care, treatment, or service, such as wraparound services, day treatment, or outpatient

---

Figure 1-2

Continuous Assessment: The Structure

Data Collection
History—Presenting Issues—Progress Notes
Physical (medical history, physical or physical health screening,
and laboratory tests)
Psychological (mental status and psychological tests)
Social (family, education, work, military, spiritual, legal, and vocational)

Action		**Assessment**
Implementation ⟷	**Individual Served** ⟷	(Evaluation)
(Interventions)		
Services, Case		
Management		

Action Planning
Care Plan Including Goals and
Objectives

This figure depicts the core elements of the assessment structure.

Source: Joint Commission Resources: *A Practical Guide to Documentation in Behavioral Health Care,* 2nd ed. Oakbrook
Terrace, IL: The Joint Commission, 2002.

---

services, the initial assessment session may be deferred until the individual's first scheduled appointment. In crisis stabilization and residential settings, the client must have a physical health assessment, including a medical history and physical examination. In all non–24-hour care settings, the client must have a physical health screening to determine the need for a physical health assessment. The physical examination or screening protects the client from life-threatening physical health problems that might be concealed because of behavioral health issues and determines whether a physical condition is contributing to the behavioral health problem or whether a physical health problem may be complicated by a behavioral health condition.

DESIGNING THE STRUCTURE OF CARE DOCUMENTATION

Regardless of the type or level of care, treatment, or service, the structure of care encompasses at least the following elements or steps:

- Intake screening/admission/assessment
- Physical and psychosocial assessment
- Analysis of data and assessments
- Prioritization of needs
- Planning of care and plan of care review/update

- Intervention (services) implementation
- Discharge/continuing planning of care

Because of the individualized manner in which the documentation processes are carried out over various organizations, the Joint Commission does not mandate the use of a specific documentation format. How these steps are implemented and documented should be organization-specific and unique to each organization's parameters. Even the names or titles of the steps may vary. For example, not every organization will use the terms *analysis of assessments, continuing plan of care,* or *psychosocial assessment.* The attributed name, title, and format are of secondary importance to the processes and outcomes. Providers are encouraged to devote greater energy to focusing on the quality of the documentation than to the aesthetics, nomenclature, or patterns of the clinical/case record forms.

The organization's mission, vision, values, philosophy, and standards of practice; the characteristics of the client; the physical environment; and the composition of an organization's staff are factors that should define the processes, the format(s), the steps, and the names of the structure and process of care. Granted, the vocabulary and content requirements of payers, including managed care, licensing bodies, and accrediting agencies, are imposing influences, but they should not determine what a process is called or its scope. First and foremost, clinical/case records should be functional for those who use them. Accordingly, Joint Commission standards emphasize the use of uniform data definitions and vocabulary for individual organizations, tailored to fit their needs. After the record is functional for the users, refinements can be made to adapt it to the requirements of payers, regulators, and accreditors. In the case of the Joint Commission's standards, specific expectations are not mandated, but principles and guiding concepts help organizations determine the kinds of components that should be in the records.

The thread that weaves the structured processes together is the progress note. Its main purpose is to communicate information about implementing the plan, how the client is progressing, and any emerging issues. Some organizations orchestrate their care, treatment, and services around documentation protocols, formats, and forms that have existed since the organization was founded. To continue to use them out of tradition or habit, regardless of their utility, can be frustrating and time consuming. The materials may have been developed by staff from the distant past to meet payer, licensing, or accreditation standards that no longer exist.

Many organizations still use the assessment tools, goal/objective formats, and plan of care review structures that were designed when individuals stayed in their programs longer than they do today. Staff members in these organizations often complain that they do not have sufficient time to complete the assessments, and the clients often do not complete many of the goals and objectives that had been established. It is imperative that organizations design the assessment and planning of care process to reflect the contemporary needs of the client, the scope of the program, and the anticipated length of stay, as well as what can reasonably be accomplished during the episode of care.

It might be a sound investment and a productive performance improvement project for providers to scrutinize the operational efficiency of their clinical/case record systems, formats, and protocols. Revising an organization's care information processes is a time-consuming project, but a reduction of documentation would be beneficial to the clients, staff, and administration.

Organizations may want to tag data elements in their forms and tools. The tag would relate the data element to the standard(s)/requirement(s) of the funding, licensing, regulatory, or accrediting body. When there is a change or revision in the standard(s)/requirement(s), the organization can quickly change or reuse their forms or tools accordingly to keep them current.

It could be particularly rewarding to review the degree of redundancy in data collection. For example, it may not be unusual for a client to be assessed by several different staff members on the same issue (such as family status). This could result in multiple pages and forms with the same information. Streamlining the kinds and repetitiveness of specific questions could be beneficial to the assessment process and allow staff the time to gain a broader and more in-depth assessment of the client. It would also reduce the client's frustration caused by being asked the same question(s) multiple times.

However, it may be necessary to review data from the assessments when the data do not fit within the overall profile. One example would be an individual who initially does not want to discuss physical/sexual abuse. When subsequent interviews indicate very low self-esteem, relationship and trust issues, and so on, a data review may be appropriate. A second example would be a young teenager who does not fit within his or her current level of functioning. Were the drug data, as presented by the teen, exaggerated or minimized for some psychological reason? Reassessment may be indicated.

Providers need to ask themselves whether forms should continue to structure the care process or should evolve from the care process. Systems are intended to be economical and utilitarian, to achieve optimal outcomes with minimal energy. The process of care should determine the format, content, and structure of documentation. Documentation should support the process of care, treatment, and services.

The Principles of Documentation

Documentation need not be viewed as a burdensome activity. It can play some important roles in an organization's structure of delivery of care, treatment, and services. Hillel Bodek, M.S.W., L.C.S.W.-R, B.C.D., a clinical social worker in both agency and private practice in New York City, and Chairperson of the Committee on Ethics and Professional Standards and of the Committee on Forensic Clinical Social Work of the New York State Society for Clinical Social Work, stresses that documentation should never be overlooked as a key component of how effectively an organization, or practitioner, delivers care. In an article directed toward the use of documentation in clinical social work, Bodek notes that legally mandated clinical documentation and record keeping serve several important purposes, most of which are equally applicable to agency and private practice settings. The clinical record has an important place in assuring the quality of clinical social work services. Professional practice standards require that clinical social work treatment be based on a proper differential diagnostic assessment and implemented in a planned manner with identified goals, methods, time frames, and criteria to measure its efficacy and appropriateness. The clinical record should document compliance with these basic practice standards.[1]

In Sidebar 1-2 on page 10, Bodek outlines what he believes are the key purposes of clinical documentation. Bodek also lists some key principles that should be kept in mind when considering clinical documentation. Although these principles were written for clinical social workers, they provide important guidelines and points for consideration for all kinds of behavioral health care settings.

DOCUMENTATION AND ORGANIZATIONAL STRUCTURE

Documentation plays a crucial role in supporting the systems and processes that deliver care, treatment, and services but can also play an important role in other areas of an organization as well, such as coding and reimbursement, resource allocation and management, and performance improvement. In addition, it is important to consider how an organization manages the privacy and security of its documents and approach to documentation.

Sidebar 1-2

Purposes of Clinical Documentation

The seven key purposes of clinical documentation are as follows:

1. **To document professional work**—to record what was done, by whom, to whom, when, where, why, and with what results; to document diagnosis and assessment, treatment/services provided, the client's clinical course and clinical decision making

2. **To serve as the basis for organization and continuity of care by the practitioner**—to record clinically meaningful information on which the practitioner can rely to refresh his or her memory of crucial events in treatment, the client's response to treatment/services, problems experienced in treatment, key historical facts and details of collateral contacts; to provide a basis for self-supervision and reflection on the client's clinical course and progress; to create a longitudinal record of the patient

3. **To serve as the basis for subsequent continuity of care by other practitioners**—to provide clinically meaningful data regarding the evaluation, treatment, progress and response to treatment, treatment planning/goals, and problems in treatment—data on which other practitioners can base decisions concerning the continuity of care/services provided to the client

4. **To provide risk management and malpractice protection**—to provide documentation of informed consent for treatment, release of records, and so on; documentation of the nature of the professional relationship and duty owed with regard to the client; documentation of professional decision making, problems encountered in working with the patient, supervision/consultation obtained, and professional response to crisis and other special situations; documentation that will support the adequacy of the clinical assessment, the appropriateness of the treatment/service plan and the application of professional skills and knowledge in the provision of professional services; substantiation of the treatment/services provided and of the results of such treatment/services

5. **To comply with legal, regulatory, and institutional requirements**—to ensure compliance with record-keeping requirements of agencies, departments, accrediting programs (for example, the Joint Commission), and third-party payers (Medicare, Workers' Compensation, Medicaid, insurance plans, and so on)

6. **To facilitate quality assurance and utilization review**—to record professional activities, purposes, and results; document appropriateness, necessity, and effectiveness of treatment/services provided; document the need for further treatment/services or to support termination of treatment/services; facilitate supervision, consultation, and staff development; help improve the quality of services by identifying problems with service delivery and providing data upon which effective corrective action can be based; provide data for educational planning, policy development, program planning, and research

7. **To facilitate coordination of professional efforts**—to facilitate communication between members of the treatment team, thereby ensuring coordinated rather than fragmented treatment/service delivery

Source: Excerpted and summarized from "Standards for Clinical Documentation and Recordkeeping," by Hillel Bodek, M.S.W., L.C.S.W.-R, B.C.D. © 2003, 2006, 2007. Used with permission. Permission to reproduce for educational purposes is granted provided attribution is included.

Coding and Reimbursement

Managing a behavioral health care organization in the current health care climate requires that systems and processes be in place to ensure that the organization is able to cover its expenses and operate viably. This translates into the need for all documentation and plans for documentation to take into consideration any coding that may be required for timely and appropriate reimbursement.

Performance Improvement

The large amounts of raw data collected in the process of documentation can help an organization's performance improvement efforts. Analysis of the aggregated data might reveal areas in need of improvement or identify staff learning needs associated with clinical care. Consider this example: Performance improvement staff in a residential addiction program review the health status reports and note an increase in client falls. A closer study of this finding by the organization determines that most of these accidents are occurring in one area of the facility and that shortly before the increase in falls began, cleaning staff had switched to a different floor-cleaning product. This product was leaving a slightly oily residue on the floors, which may have contributed to the increase in falls. The organization decides to change the cleaning product and add additional safety measures around the facility. Shortly thereafter, the rate of client falls is reduced significantly.

Resource Allocation and Management

Although not all documentation in an organization will relate specifically to the provision of care, treatment, and services, it can and does support it. The use of effective documentation should not be limited to the realm of clinical documentation alone. For example, many behavioral health care organizations use resources and equipment that play a primary role in that organization's delivery of care, treatment, and services, and how they manage the documentation about that maintenance and usage can have an impact on how effectively their organization functions and how well it provides care to the populations it serves.

One example is the case of VisionQuest, a youth services organization, and how one of its key programs—equine excursions—is maintained and tracked. VisionQuest has determined that not providing a system to track and maintain the horses that play a pivotal role in one of its outdoor programs can have an impact on client safety and effective resource management. Sidebar 1-3 on pages 12–13 shares VisionQuest's process to manage and maintain its equine resources.

THE CHANGING WORLD OF DOCUMENTATION
Security and Privacy Issues in Documentation

The Joint Commission's documentation-related standards for behavioral health care apply to both paper-based and computerized records. In both cases, special consideration must be given to how those records are secured and maintained. For instance, security of electronic clinical/case records needs to be clearly defined for both those who have access to the records and those who have the ability to enter or revise data in that record. In the case of paper-based documentation, the location, access, and protection of the records must be determined and carefully protected. The standards on confidentiality and security are applicable.

Privacy and the protection of clients is driven by the Health Insurance Portability and Accountability Act (HIPAA) and its Privacy Rule, which went into effect in 2003. Organizations need to take measures to ensure that their documentation and how it is managed fits within the parameters of HIPAA and ensures the privacy of the client while ensuring that the case/clinical record

Sidebar 1-3

Managing the Documentation of Resources

VisionQuest is a national youth services organization that provides intervention services to at-risk youth and families. In existence since the early 1970s, it offers residential and other services for at-risk youth in Arizona, California, Delaware, Pennsylvania, New Jersey, Florida, and Maryland. One program offered since almost the inception of VisionQuest is the use of equine-assisted therapy. Skilled instructors use natural horse training as a means by which to teach important life skills. Another program offered is the "wagon train" in which youth travel cross-country on horseback and via covered wagon. As a result, VisionQuest has amassed a significant resource in its horses, which it maintains and tracks at different facilities throughout the country. The well-being and effective use of these horses plays a pivotal role in the effectiveness of the equine excursions, so VisionQuest has devised some systems to help it ensure that operations run smoothly.

Dennis Call, risk manager for the Adventure Program at VisionQuest, has been working with the equine staff to develop a tracking system that ensures that the program is safe, the horses are well cared for and appropriately inventoried, the gear is safe and up-to-date, and the staff are able to effectively serve the youth through this program. "We have approximately 80 horses throughout the country right now, and we developed the system to ensure that we are using the same, consistent manner in how we track and maintain our equine services," Call notes.

Before launching the new system, VisionQuest's various horse stations around the country did not always operate in the same way and did not always collect the same data on each horse. By establishing a consistent system, Call is now able to track the status of each horse, any accidents or near misses on every excursion, and how well the gear for the horses is being maintained. As they are transferred between facilities, each horse carries a comprehensive record that includes its history, vaccinations, transfer information, any additional veterinary or medical information and any changes in status. Because it travels with each horse, the permanent record is not difficult to locate when information is needed. Each facility also maintains its own log and inventory of equipment. (*See* Figures 1-3 through 1-7 on the companion CD-ROM for examples of these forms.) The forms provide VisionQuest with a comprehensive picture of the horse, its location, the gear used for it, and any transfers undertaken. "All the contents of the horse's file are placed in order as listed on the Equine Inventory Sheet (*see* Figure 1-3) to bring uniformity," explains Call. "We use the transfer record (*see* Figure 1-7) frequently as our animals are transferred between geographical locations according to season, activities and events, and census. This form gives us a history if we need to track information on health or behavior issues."

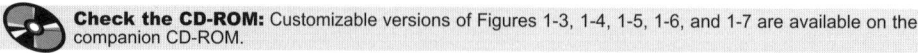 **Check the CD-ROM:** Customizable versions of Figures 1-3, 1-4, 1-5, 1-6, and 1-7 are available on the companion CD-ROM.

Each horse facility is also responsible for maintaining its own documentation on gear repairs and inventory. This plays an important role in ensuring that there are no added risks during a wagon trail or other equine-related therapy. "It is impossible to ensure that nothing will ever happen during one of these excursions," notes Call. "Sometimes a horse will have a reaction that you can't predict, or the trail will cause a problem. But there are some things we can do to help mitigate the risks." Call points to taking a careful inventory of gear as an example of this. "We can lessen the risks significantly by ensuring that our equipment is working properly, so we have put some checks into the process to help us with that."

(continued)

Sidebar 1-3 (continued)

Staff at the various horse stations also submit information to Call on a regular basis so he can track the horses and equipment to see if any actions need to be taken. For example, it may be determined that a particular horse needs to be rotated out of regular use in order to rest or that a specific piece of gear needs updating.

Getting staff on board with the new system took some time and effort, but now that it is being used regularly, it has become part of normal operations. "Our horse staff doesn't typically have a lot of background in documentation, but with some training and mentoring they are all using the system, and we have left the process open so we can make changes or improvements should it be warranted." Call opted to create a series of forms that are functional yet able to be updated in case the organization finds that it wants to make changes. Call acknowledges that the organization could have spent more time finessing or formalizing the forms before it began using them, but he finds that the best way to determine the viability of certain documentation is to use it and make modifications if needed.

Call has found that keeping a consistent system of collecting and reporting data works very well for all of the adventure programs that VisionQuest offers. "We had the case some time ago where I was receiving reports on several bike accidents happening in one of our outdoor programs over a short period of time," he explains. "Once I saw this trend, I started to investigate and found that the accidents were happening at the same point on the bike ride." Call did some additional research and determined that this particular bend in the route was close to the end of the ride and that the young bikers were most likely being more reckless in their riding style because they saw that they were nearing the end of the ride.

"To deal with this we changed the layout of the ride to have a less difficult turn toward the end and also gave youth the option of dismounting and pushing their bikes through for the last part of the ride," Call explains. Using and analyzing the available data and responding quickly allowed VisionQuest to reduce the risk on its bike rides. And having a consistent and widespread approach to documentation has helped the organization provide services to its young clients while eliminating as much risk as possible.

---

is as complete as possible. In the case of some types of documentation—such as "psychotherapy notes"—it must be kept separate from the actual case record due to the highly private nature of the material. HIPAA mandates that this information "be kept to a higher standard of protection because they are not part of the medical record and are never intended to be shared with anyone else." Various states also have confidentiality laws regarding clinical information. There is also a federal confidentiality law for substance abuse treatment.*

While privileged and private information, such as psychotherapy notes, must be kept separate from the record, the vast majority of information—that which helps ensure continuity of care for a

---

* The federal confidentiality of substance abuse patient records statute, section 543 of the Public Health Service Act, 42 U.S.C. 290dd-2, and its implementing regulation, 42 CFR Part 2, establish confidentiality requirements for patient records that are maintained in connection with the performance of any federally assisted specialized alcohol or drug abuse program. Substance abuse programs are generally programs or personnel that provide alcohol or drug abuse treatment, diagnosis, or referral for treatment. The term *federally assisted* is broadly defined and includes federally conducted or funded programs, federally licensed or certified programs, and programs that are tax exempt. Certain exceptions apply to information held by the Department of Veterans Affairs and the Armed Forces.

client who has been transferred, discharged, or referred to another health care provider—must be held within the same record.

Electronic Records Versus Paper-Based Records

The technology of electronic clinical/case records is developing at a rapid pace. Some organizations have made the move toward electronic records or the use of online forms, others are using a combination of electronic and paper documentation, while others still rely exclusively on paper-based documentation. Whatever the approach may be, organizations must ensure that their method suits the needs of their staff and clients and is manageable.

Computerized or electronic records can play an important role in helping organizations with the systemization and organization of their records, but they will not resolve the critical issue of individualizing problem statements and writing centered on the needs of the client. Regardless of the format used, the imperative for accurate and complete information remains. Computers may generate documents more quickly than humans, but as with paper-based records, the quality of the information contained in an electronic record is only as good as what has been entered into it.

Systems for the use of electronic records must be appropriate to the type of care, treatment, and service offered by the organization. An organization that is considering moving toward an electronic record system should consult national behavioral health care associations or other similar organizations in their region or local area to learn what approaches are working well for others in the field.

Another recent innovation in documentation is the development of standardized forms and documentation for use by organizations within a specific region or state. One such example is the Solutions for Ohio's Quality Improvement and Compliance (SOQIC). SOQIC is a collaborative venture between the Ohio Department of Mental Health, the Ohio Department of Alcohol and Drug Addiction Services, mental health boards, providers, and clients in the state of Ohio. One outcome of the venture was the design, development, and implementation of a standardized integrated medical records forms toolset that covers the entire treatment process from demographic information to transfer/discharge, including assessment, treatment planning, and progress notes. The forms accommodate the various certification, national accreditation, and Medicare/Medicaid compliance requirements, as well as Ohio state agencies' own rules and standards. Organizations within Ohio can gain access to these tools and forms and are given the option of using either the online system or printing out paper forms.[2] This is intended to provide organizations with a low-cost and effective way of accessing and using documentation to assist with the delivery of safe, high-quality care, treatment, and services. By using such standardized forms that integrate all possible requirements and regulations, organizations can be sure that their material is not only accurate but that it meets the needs of their particular region. This move by the state of Ohio to introduce a standardized system is being considered in other states as well, including Massachusetts, Arkansas, and Michigan. Organizations should check with their own state department of mental health to determine if any similar initiative may be under consideration.

SUMMARY

Quality documentation is an essential tool in the behavioral health care workplace. It is vital to the organizational need for improved accountability. A system of any kind, whether it is for building cars or providing behavioral health care, requires continuous feedback loops to evaluate outcomes and processes so that any unacceptable performance can be detected promptly and restored to acceptable standards of practice. The clinical/case record is one such resource and is a primary database for care performance and outcome evaluation.

Each step in the care process has equal merit. There is no hierarchy within the care process, as each step builds on its predecessor. The quality of the intake/admission assessment affects the quality of the continuing plan of care. If an intake assessment fails to detect or omits important information, each subsequent step in the care process is affected. Performance expectations for any single step have parity with any other. The process of care is seamless, dynamic, and cumulative. What occurs at the end is dependent on what has occurred from the initial point of contact onward.

Documentation should be a movie of the client: How was he or she on arrival, what happened during the time in care, and how was he or she upon discharge or transfer? It should provide a three-dimensional living guide to that client instead of a two-dimensional snapshot. It should include the catalytic guideposts for care, treatment, and services.

Only rarely is inadequate documentation a result of staff indifference. Resistance to documentation is more likely an outgrowth of insufficient or inadequate staff training. Few people look forward to assuming tasks for which they have not been adequately prepared. Everyone enjoys doing what they do well. Practical, utilitarian skill building should enhance competence.

If providers are advised that their clinical/case record entries can be simple and realistic, their dread of documentation tasks may disappear. Training to improve documentation skills has become a high priority as clinical/service and administrative leaders more fully recognize the relationship between quality case recording and organization performance. Improved clinical/case record documentation improves organization performance because it does the following:

- Enables the client to actively and knowledgeably participate in his or her plan of care, treatment, or service
- Manages care, treatment, or services
- Enhances organization finances by reducing denied reimbursement claims
- Establishes a database for the organization to evaluate and improve performance
- Enables leaders to allocate their time and resources efficiently
- Establishes a database to improve staff competence

The enhancement of documentation skills is a sound investment for organizational leadership. The return on investment is shared by both the client and providers.

REFERENCES

1. Bodek, H.: *Standards for Clinical Documentation and Recordkeeping.* New York State Society for Clinical Social Work. http://www.clinicalsw.org/basic_standards.html (accessed Sep. 15, 2007).
2. Ohio Department of Mental Health: *SOQIC: A New Standard in Documentation.* http://www.mh.state.oh.us/cmtymh/soqic/soqic.index.html (accessed Sep. 15, 2007).

Section 2

THE PROCESS AND STRUCTURE OF SCREENING/ASSESSMENT

Assessment is an ongoing activity that dominates the care process. Each interaction with a client requires assimilating information, weighing it, responding to its meaning, and again assimilating information regarding the client's response. It is one of the most important functions within the continuum of care, treatment, and services. Although data collection is a significant part of the assessment process, it is not synonymous with it. Data collection serves as the foundation, but the evaluation of the data is the linchpin. Reporting data without evaluation represents only partial completion of the assessment process.

Teachers maintain that the best learning comes from personal experience. However, it is also possible to benefit from the experience of others. For most of us, it is less threatening and embarrassing to ponder the errors of others than to make them ourselves. This chapter gives examples of opportunities for documentation improvement experienced by others and offers recommendations to facilitate improvement.

The first step in ensuring that documentation is well prepared and serves the needs of the organization is to keep sound guiding principles in mind whenever preparing it. Consider the following qualities that can comprise good documentation[1]:

- Provides relevant information in appropriate detail
- Is organized with appropriate headings and logical progression
- Is thoughtful, reflecting the application of professional knowledge, skills, and judgment in the treatment/services provided
- Is appropriately concise
- Serves the purposes of documentation (as outlined above) that are applicable to a given situation
- Uses relevant direct quotes from the client and from other sources
- Distinguishes clearly between facts, observations, hard data, and opinions
- States the source(s) of the facts, observations, hard data, opinions, and other information being relied upon, and provides an assessment of the reliability of this material
- Is internally consistent
- Is written in the present tense, as appropriate

Sidebar 2-1, pages 18–20, identifies terms used in this chapter and briefly defines them. Care providers may use different language to describe or define the same terms.

Sidebar 2-1

Documentation Terms

Analysis of significant data: The analysis consolidates the significant information gathered from all assessments of the client into a single evaluation. The analysis ensures that when a portion of an assessment focuses on a single aspect of the life of the client (physical or psychosocial), the information is then integrated with all the other aspects. When done effectively, the analysis will allow evaluation and prioritization of the needs and strengths of the client.

The Joint Commission considers the analysis of data to be a process, not a specific document. Therefore, providers do not have to develop a separate document if another document or process blends the separate physical and psychosocial findings into a whole portrait of the client.

Providers are required to consider information obtained by each discipline that played a part in the assessment of the client and then analyze and prioritize the needs of the client while developing the plan of care. This process may be performed during a team meeting, if that is the structure of the organization, and reflected in a progress note or meeting minutes. Other methods include a synthesized assessment and/or plan of care, discharge plan, or problems/needs list.

Cultural/ethnic assessment: A cultural/ethnic assessment evaluates the cultural influences on the existing value system of the client and how cultural/ethnic influences affect the conditions that bring him or her to care, treatment, or service. Cultural influences include ethnicity, race, gender, geography, and socioeconomic status.

Emotional and behavioral assessment: The evaluation of the emotional, behavioral, and cognitive functioning of the client is conducted by a variety of professionals who have been deemed competent to conduct such assessments by virtue of licensure and/or organizational standards. It is conducted at the time of intake and continuously thereafter during care, treatment, or service. It includes an evaluation of the following:
- Current emotional and behavioral functioning
- History of emotional and behavioral problems and/or treatment
- Family history of psychological problems
- Cognitive functioning
- Maladaptive or problem behaviors
- History of addictive behaviors by client or by family members, such as drug abuse or gambling
- Emotional and behavioral functioning

Physical assessment: In 24-hour settings, physicians and nursing personnel (or a community source) may conduct the evaluation of the physical needs of the client. This includes a medical history and physical examination. (*Note:* The physical assessment will also include review and evaluation of any applicable laboratory work requested as part of the physical examination.) In crisis stabilization and acute care settings, the physical assessment is completed within 24 hours. In residential programs, the assessment is completed within 1 week.

For children, youth, and persons with developmental disabilities, the physical assessment should also include an evaluation of the following:
- Motor development and functioning

(continued)

Sidebar 2-1 (continued)

- Sensorimotor functioning
- Speech, hearing, and language functioning
- Oral health and hygiene
- Visual functioning
- Immunization status

In opioid treatment programs the physical assessment is completed within 14 days. In all other types of non–24-hour care organizations, a screening to determine the need for a physical examination is required. Any screening tools that these providers use need to be designed with input from a qualified and competent licensed independent practitioner.

Psychosocial assessment: This assessment consists of the evaluation of psychological and social functioning of the client, including conflicts or problems involving the following:
- Environment and living situation
- Leisure and recreation
- Religious and spiritual orientation
- Childhood history
- Military service history
- Financial issues
- Usual social, peer group, and environmental setting
- Sexual history
- Family circumstances
- Mental status (when indicated)
- Psychiatric evaluation (when indicated)
- Psychological evaluation (when indicated)
- History of previous behavioral problems and/or care, treatment, or service

The evaluation also includes determining the appropriateness and level of need for inclusion of the family of the client.

Spiritual assessment: Part of the psychosocial assessment but not required for all settings. The spiritual assessment evaluates such factors as the philosophical orientation of the client toward the purpose and meaning of life and his or her relationship with humanity (degree of isolation, degree of alienation from others) or a higher power. It is not solely intended to identify the religion or religious practices of the client, but to analyze how (if at all) the spiritual orientation of the client affects his or her lifestyle.

Practice guidelines: Descriptive tools or standardized specifications for care of the typical client in the typical situation, developed through a formal process that incorporates the best scientific evidence of effectiveness with expert opinion. Synonyms include practice parameters, preferred practice patterns, and guidelines.

(continued)

Sidebar 2-1 (continued)

Problems/needs list: A formal, written problems or needs list is not required by The Joint Commission. However, as a result of the completion of the data collection and assessment, the provider should be aware of all the problems or deficits of the client. These will be sorted into three groups: problems for which care, treatment, or service will be provided; problems to be deferred; and problems for which referral is indicated. These three groups constitute the problems/needs list. This may be a written list or merely the conceptualization of the prioritized care needs of the client. This is the process that leads to the "clinical or case formulation." Again, these may be written or demonstrated through a comprehensive plan of care. The end result is prioritization of care, either through a comprehensive plan of care, a case conference, or other process.

Strength assessment: Strength assessments are good practice but are not required by the Joint Commission. A strengths-based assessment identifies the positive resources and abilities in clients. Strength-based assessment is "the measurement of emotional and behavioral skills, competencies, and characteristics that create a sense of personal accomplishment; contribute to satisfying relationships with family members, peers, and adults; enhance one's ability to deal with adversity and stress; and promote one's personal, social, and academic development."[2]

USING HISTORY AND DATA COLLECTION AS THE FOUNDATION FOR EVALUATION

Restating the history and data of the client in abbreviated form rather than evaluating them is the most widespread documentation error in behavioral health care and human service programs. When providers discuss clients, they include a plethora of evaluative statements. They draw inferences about the behavior of clients based on the information they have collected; however, when they then write what is called an assessment, they often limit their narrative to a mere repetition of data. Although data serve as background material, they do not alone constitute evaluation.

EXAMPLE A 30-year-old woman enters a local mental health center complaining of fatigue and an inability to perform normal daily tasks. Most days she does not get dressed or leave the house. This behavior began three years ago, shortly after her only child died in an automobile accident. She states that she has used alcohol and prescription medication to cope. However, it seems that the situation has become more severe, and her alcohol and drug use has increased. The client might be considered a "mentally ill chemical abuser" (MICA) because the following criteria of that classification are present:

- Chronic or long-standing symptoms that fit into a diagnostic category, such as depression
- Chemical use to the point that there is a negative impact on the client's ability to function—a pathological use of alcohol and drugs
- Both disorders have existed over a long period of time.
- There is significant functional impairment in areas such as self-care and socialization.

Perhaps the only further consideration is to ensure that a staff person with experience and competence in MICA provides care for this client. This will be necessary to determine whether her inability to care for herself is a factor in the mental illness, chemical use, or both.

However, consider the issues that are discovered when a comprehensive assessment is completed. First, in reviewing the treatment, care, and service history of this client, clinicians learn that when she was 17, she received treatment for a year after becoming abnormally withdrawn. Her family history indicates that both her mother and her sister have treatment histories, and that her sister has a history of suicide attempts. Upon further review, it is determined that the client has also considered suicide and has stockpiled prescription medication in the past. In an assessment of physical or sexual abuse, the client specifies that her father sexually abused her when she was between the ages of 13 and 16. In reviewing the history and patterns of alcohol and substance abuse, it is determined that she began using alcohol at age 16 and has used on a daily basis since age 17. She began drinking two or three beers a day, but now drinks a pint of vodka daily. In the physical assessment she indicates that she frequently goes for days without eating.

Analysis of data collected has indicated priorities for care and further assessment. Now consider the impact if the behavioral health care professional's summary had followed these lines:

"You are a 30-year-old Caucasian female. You are married and have had one child who is deceased. You live at home with your spouse. You are not employed. Your family has a history of mental illness; your mother and sister were treated on an outpatient basis; and you have a history of psychiatric treatment. You deny any leisure or recreational activities or interests. You deny any military history. Your nutritional history is poor and you have a 13-year history of alcohol and drug abuse. Schedule an appointment for next month and we will prepare a plan of care."

Hopefully, in the real world, no behavioral health care professional would give such a report, nor would anyone tolerate it without demanding an evaluation of all the data. This example is used to emphasize the point that reporting data is not the same as interpreting them. Unfortunately, the caricature mimics what is often identified in clinical/case records as an assessment. It is an unfortunate example of the most commonly found documentation error: the failure to evaluate data.

There is a wealth of information in the behavioral health care professional's report, but none of it is evaluated. The narrative lacks any appraisal or evaluation of what the data mean for that client. Histories and data can be very similar for different clients, but their behavioral consequences, or outcomes, have infinite variability because of the unique characteristics of each client. For example, the backgrounds and histories of adolescents in care programs can be remarkably similar, but behavioral outcomes and consequences distinguish one teenager from another. The alcohol and drug history of any client in an addiction program can be similar to the histories of other clients in the same program. Again, it is the individualized meaning and consequences of the history that distinguish one person with an addictive behavior from another.

Thus, although taking a history and collecting data are critical activities, the evaluation and interpretation of data determine and define the need for care and its processes. Evaluation and interpretation constitute the pillars of assessment. Simply reducing a four-page history to a one-page history is creating a synopsis, not an assessment. It is the individualized meaning, consequences, and outcomes of assessment data that distinguish one client from another.

In the previous example, the data were relevant to the client and should have been shared with her. But from the client's perspective, there was even more critical information that was not communicated. It might have been communicated by responding to certain questions, such as the following:

- What do all these data mean?
- What is my condition?
- What are my problems?
- What have I been doing that I should continue to do?
- What should I do to maintain my health and to resolve the problems I have, and how do I begin?
- What can you or others do to help me?
- What can I do to help myself?
- What should I look for and watch to see if I am progressing?

Questions such as these constitute a major portion of clinical assessment, but can be missing from the records of clients.

In actual practice, the behavioral health care professional would address these issues as follows:

- "We need to further assess issues or thoughts concerning suicide. We need to help you stay safe."
- "We want to further evaluate the trauma that occurred when you were 16 and also the trauma from the death of your child."
- "We want to initiate further evaluation of your physical health to identify problems that may have been caused by poor nutritional habits and alcohol and drug abuse."
- "Finally, we want to address the alcohol and drug abuse issue and your depression."

Unfortunately, some providers do not write assessments that are as detailed and complete as when an assessment is discussed verbally—that is, when the discussion is more of an evaluation. It is not that providers fail to complete evaluations or to identify questions, but that they sometimes do not write them proficiently and sometimes do not write them at all. Instead, they write mini-histories. It can really benefit the process of documentation and planning if staff take time to write precise, detailed documentation that mirrors much of what is said verbally.

THE ASSESSMENT

The primary areas of assessment addressed in this book are physical functioning and psychosocial functioning.

Categorizing the various assessments under physical or psychosocial aspects can seem arbitrary. This categorization does not imply which discipline needs to perform which aspect. For instance, in many outpatient programs a single provider (such as a social worker) completes the entire assessment, including the health screening and psychosocial aspects. Before establishing assessment formats and processes, providers should review the requirements that they are expected to meet from payers, regulators, and accreditors, and they should be aware of their organization's mission and scope of services, as well as the population(s) served.

In Sidebar 2-2 on pages 23–25, Hillel Bodek, M.S.W., L.C.S.W.-R, B.C.D., (see Section 1) shares what elements should be included in an appropriate initial assessment and treatment plan. Although this has been written primarily with the clinical social worker in mind, the principles outlined in the sidebar should be taken into consideration for other kinds of behavioral health care settings.

Sidebar 2-2

Elements of an Appropriate Initial Assessment and Treatment Plan

An initial differential diagnostic assessment, which may be abbreviated or elongated depending on the circumstances of a particular case, provides the basis for the development and implementation of the treatment plan. As with any other area of clinical practice, lack of proper clinical assessment is likely to result in less than optimal and perhaps inadequate or inappropriate treatment. Thus, the failure to conduct an appropriate differential diagnostic assessment or to develop an appropriate treatment plan is a serious deviation from the standard of care owed by a clinical social worker to a client. The conduct and documentation of a proper initial assessment, and the development of an initial treatment plan includes the following:

1. Identification of the referral source(s), gathering information about the background and reasons for the referral, and assessing the client's response to and expectations regarding the referral

2. Defining the presenting problem(s), both in the client's own words using appropriate quotations, as well as in terms of the clinician's perception of the presenting problem(s)

3. Detailing the history and clinical course of the presenting problem(s) and the details of services and treatment the client has sought or received to deal with those problems

4. Gathering and documenting relevant history from the client and from collateral sources, in appropriate detail, by topic, identifying the sources of such historical information assessing the reliability of the information, regarding the following:

   a. Family history, including a list of family members in families of origin and procreation and basic demographic information about them (for example, birthplace, education, occupation, age, and cause of death, if applicable), a brief description about their relationship with the client, marital history, and any family history of mental, neurological, substance abuse/alcoholism, or serious medical problems

   b. Medical history, including serious or chronic ailments, hospitalizations, serious physical trauma, surgery, allergies, any chronic medications, and all current medications, including over-the-counter drugs, supplements, herbs, and other alternative treatments

   c. Psychiatric history, including mental health symptoms and treatment, hospitalizations (including whether voluntary or not), response to previous mental health treatment (including response to and side effects of particular psychotropic medications that have been prescribed), previous psychotherapy and client's response to and feelings about therapy, history of treatment compliance and noncompliance, and, if client left treatment, why he or she did so

   d. History of alcohol and other substance abuse and alcoholism and substance abuse treatment, including, for each substance of abuse (including alcohol), the substance, the first and most recent use of the substance, the method(s) of use, the amount used/time period (for example, $10 of crack/day, five 40 oz. bottles of beer/weekend, and so on), the frequency of use (steady on a daily basis, binging once every three or four weeks for one to three days, and so on), the duration of use, any significant periods of abstinence (including how these were achieved and why they ended), the social context of the substance abuse (alone, sharing with others, only at parties), identified triggers for the

(continued)

Sidebar 2-2 (continued)

substance abuse, treatment programs attended (which ones, when, and for how long; did the client complete the program successfully, and if not, why?), and biopsychosocial impact of the substance abuse on the client

e. Child and adolescent developmental history, including family and peer group relationships, home life, socioeconomic status, schooling, parenting and discipline, type of neighborhood and housing, learning disabilities and other developmental delays; in children and young adolescents a more detailed developmental history is usually indicated

f. Educational history, including level of academic achievement, academic strengths and weaknesses, relationships with teachers, history of being denied regular promotion, placement in special education or other special educational programs, school behavior (including any suspensions, expulsions, or school transfers)

g. History of occupational training/skills and work history, including significant employment, work-related difficulties, general salary information, and adult economic status

h. History of interpersonal relationships, nature and extent of peer group relationships, and nature and type of significant interpersonal problems

i. History of past and current social support systems, including the impact of these, or the lack of these, on the client's development and functioning

j. Juvenile and criminal justice history, including the nature of any arrests, convictions, and sentences imposed; and history of patterns of antisocial behavior

k. History of sexual relationships or psychosexual problems and issues, including sexual orientation and sexual dysfunction

l. History of religious affiliation and practices and issues relating to religion

m. Racial, cultural, ethnic, and nationality issues

n. History of physical, emotional, or sexual abuse or other victimization from the client and from collateral sources, in appropriate detail, by topic, identifying the sources of such historical information and assessing the reliability of the information

5. Describing the practitioner's observations of the client, the results of a mental status examination, an assessment of the client's strengths and weaknesses or limitations, and gathering information about the client's general physical health (including any current or recent symptoms or health problems and any current or recent health care treatment)

6. Detailing previous clinical services, the background and reasons for which those services were sought and provided, the results of such services, and the reason(s) for termination of those services

7. Making a differential biopsychosocial diagnosis using all five DSM-IV axes, and an assessment of the patient in functional as well as diagnostic terms, which distinguishes between observations, hard data, and opinions; sets forth the support for generalizations and conclusions in the assessment; and makes a determination about the clinician's degree of confidence in the assessment

8. An assessment of whether the client poses a risk of decompensation, suicidality, assaultiveness, homicidality, relapse back to alcoholism or substance abuse, inability to care for himself or herself, risk of being victimized, of victimizing others, or is at any other serious risk; include the basis for the risk assessment, details of the steps taken at intake to address any of these risks, and the results of those steps

(continued)

Sidebar 2-2 (continued)

9. Developing an initial differential treatment or service plan with identified long-term goals and short-term objectives, methods to be used, time frames and standards to measure treatment progress in functional terms, with a rationale for prioritizing treatment goals and for the choice from among various treatment alternatives and strategies. The plan may include services from other providers, in which case these should be identified by function and/or name, and the services to be provided by them specified.

10. An assessment of prognosis with supporting rationale

11. Describing the client's response to the assessment and to the proposed treatment plan and, if the client agrees to proceed with that plan, documenting informed consent for implementation of that plan.

Source: Excerpted and summarized from "Standards for Clinical Documentation and Recordkeeping," by Hillel Bodek, M.S.W., L.C.S.W.-R, B.C.D. © 2003, 2006, 2007. Used with permission. Permission to reproduce for educational purposes is granted provided attribution is included.

Physical Assessments

The Joint Commission requires that a physical health assessment, including a medical history and physical examination, be completed within 24 hours after admission to inpatient or crisis stabilization programs and within 1 week after admission to residential programs.

All non–24-hour care programs (as well as shelters, supportive living, case management, and assertive community treatment) need to develop written procedures requiring a physical health screening to determine the need for a physical health assessment, including a medical history and physical examination. Many organizations have found it beneficial to seek the assistance of a physician in developing a screening tool that can easily identify conditions that would trigger a prompt consultation. The tool may consist of a comprehensive questionnaire similar to those used in physicians' offices. It may consist of a telephone consultation with a physician. Whatever the approved mechanism, it must be implemented and documented in the clinical/case record.

> The health screening includes at least the following:
> - Past and current diagnoses, problems, or conditions
> - Significant past care, treatment, or service procedures
> - Known adverse and allergic drug reactions
> - Currently and recently used medications

For foster care children, medical history and physical examinations are performed in an appropriate time frame to comply with laws and regulations, and within a time frame that accommodates the best interests and welfare of the child.

> The Joint Commission's standards do not mandate formats or content for the physical health assessment except for the following populations:
> - Children
> - Youth
> - Persons with developmental disabilities
>
> For these populations, the physical assessment must include the following:
> - Motor development and functioning
> - Sensorimotor functioning
> - Speech, hearing, and language functioning
> - Visual functioning
> - Immunization status
> - Oral health/hygiene

Persons with developmental disabilities require at least annual assessments of physical development, developmental history, and health.

If the comprehensive medical history and physical examinations have been completed within 30 days of a client's admission, a legible copy of the information can be substituted, provided that any changes (or no changes) in the client's condition since it was completed are recorded. By inference, it would appear that a primary care provider would have to document the review of the physical information, evaluate the client's condition, and determine whether further assessments are warranted.

In Sidebar 2-3 on pages 27–28, one residential program shares its experience with using both an initial health screening and subsequent physical assessment for the new clients admitted to its program.

Screening/Assessment

Some assessment aspects in the Joint Commission standards require organizations to "determine the need to assess" or perform assessments "when indicated."

"As needed" assessments include the following:
- Functional status (including physical, language, self-care, visual-motor, cognitive)
- Mental status examination
- Psychiatric evaluation
- Psychological
- Community resources accessed by the client
- Vocational
- Educational
- Physical health (in non–24-hour care settings)

Criteria for making referrals to select aspects/disciplines need to be identified and documented in policies/plans by each organization. Organizations are strongly encouraged to include appropriate providers to develop or approve referral criteria (that is, a qualified psychologist needs to approve the criteria used to prompt a referral for a psychological evaluation, and a qualified social worker needs to approve the criteria used to prompt a referral for a social assessment).

Sidebar 2-3

Physical Assessment and Screening in a Residential Program

For behavioral health care organizations, ensuring that the information collected at admission is timely, thorough, and appropriate for the needs of the clients they serve can be challenging. Further, the plan of care for a client must be created as quickly as possible. VisionQuest, an at-risk youth intervention program with residential, nonresidential, and outdoor programs, works to have a full understanding of the needs and issues of each youth, but also must be sure that the youth are physically well enough to participate in the program. As a result, VisionQuest has designed an assessment process that helps the organization obtain the most thorough information as quickly as possible. "You want to hit the ground running," explains Nancy Plerhoples, A.C.S.W., national accreditation manager, for VisionQuest.

"While it's impossible to get all of the right information as quickly as possible all of the time, our assessment and screening forms are designed to help us be as effective as possible," Plerhoples continues. In the case of its residential programs, Plerhoples explains that VisionQuest will not clear any youth for participation in the outdoor programs until their physical assessment is complete.

"Our primary work takes place in outdoor settings and the youth must be able to participate. So we want to get a sense of their physical well-being and any history items that we need to be aware of," Plerhoples explains. The screening and assessment includes ensuring general health, dealing with or accommodating any chronic or treated conditions, and ensuring that the youth undergo additional physical examination with a physician, if warranted.

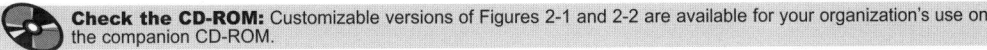

Check the CD-ROM: Customizable versions of Figures 2-1 and 2-2 are available for your organization's use on the companion CD-ROM.

When a youth is admitted, VisionQuest uses a screening form (*see* Figure 2-1 on CD-ROM) to rule out specific high-risk health concerns, such as tuberculosis, and to determine what degree of additional assessment or treatment may be warranted. The form itself will help trigger certain types of responses as well. For example, if the screener determines that the youth has a high fever, the organization requires that the youth be isolated from the general population until medically evaluated. The form also deals with screening for such issues as addictions or suicide risk and triggers an appropriate response. At the end of the two-page form, the screener is asked to select the next step for the youth. This is signed by multiple staff at the organization and initiates the next step in the process.

Youth determined not to have any evident health issues will be joined to the general population but will still (like all of the youth admitted) undergo an additional and more comprehensive health and safety evaluation plan (*see* Figure 2-2 on CD-ROM), typically the next step in the assessment process for admitted youth. This form is part assessment and part treatment planning in nature and allows care providers at the organization to delve deeper into any health or safety issues to help determine the type of plan of care needed. It also provides a single document for the organization to record findings about the youth and any plan of care that is put in place.

The first four pages of the health and safety evaluation form are generally completed by way of interview and examination with the youth. After the form is completed, staff will determine a preliminary plan of care. A multidisciplinary group work together to develop and implement the plan.

Plerhoples sees great safety benefits and risk reduction potential in a thorough use of these forms upon admission. "I think that when the forms are done carefully, the goal is to prevent problems," she explains. "Our emphasis is on prevention. We want to make sure that we have as complete a picture

(continued)

Sidebar 2-3 (continued)

of each individual as possible and that youth understand the need for safety. Our goal in all of our programs is to have no physical restraint. So right off the bat we ask youth what can we do to help them act safely." And having a comprehensive process of both screening and assessment has helped VisionQuest effectively focus on the work of healing for the youth it serves.

When considering designing new forms or making updates or changes to existing ones, Plerhoples offers the following suggestions:

✓ *Involve health care front-line staff.* Don't forget to involve your staff who use the forms on a regular basis or who might be asked to start using the new form. If you are modifying existing forms, ask them what has been problematic in the form and what works well. Also tap into their expertise to help you develop the forms. Ask them what they think you should include.

✓ *Make sure you know your regulations.* To keep the process of documentation as streamlined and simple as possible, make sure that whatever forms you use or develop take into consideration all requirements and expectations from regulating agencies or accrediting organizations. It can save time and work to keep things in one place.

✓ *Always keep the population you serve in mind.* When you develop any material it should always be specifically developed for the population you are serving. There are no "cookie cutter" forms to use. Always ask if the form meets the needs of the population and if it provides the needed information.

✓ *Be creative and think outside the box.* Some of the innovations in documentation that VisionQuest developed over the years has been due to having to "think on their feet." Due to the nature of the kinds of programs that VisionQuest offers (outdoors and often in remote locations), the organization has found that being creative and thinking outside the box has helped it develop and implement materials that have been beneficial to its ongoing work.

Screening for Pain

The first step in pain management is to screen for the existence of physical pain during a client's initial assessment. Screens detect the presence of a condition. An assessment is conducted only after pain is determined to exist. Assessment defines the type, cause, intensity, and source of pain to determine a course of treatment. If screening indicates physical pain, the organization can then do one of three things: refer the client for assessment and treatment; assess the pain and refer for treatment; or assess and treat the pain.

Several methods of pain screening or assessment should be considered in behavioral health care programs. The client may indicate pain during his or her assessment, and it should be treated or referred for assessment and/or treatment. The client may describe his or her pain in a manner that indicates a psychiatric symptom versus a physical issue. Nevertheless, reports of pain should not be ignored. Mental illness does not mean physical illness will not occur.

Finally, as in alcohol and drug programs, the withdrawal from alcohol and drugs can cause real pain. Although the withdrawal is a positive factor, the pain is still present and should be treated. Figure 2-3, *see* the companion CD-ROM, provides an example of one organization's pain assessment questionnaire for clients. In this pain assessment questionnaire, clients are encouraged to express their level of pain or discomfort in simple and straightforward terms.

Check the CD-ROM: A customizable version of Figure 2-3 is available for your organization's use on the companion CD-ROM.

Often, physical assessments indicate a need for laboratory tests, such as a blood sample drawn and sent to the laboratory for evaluation. A documented evaluation and explanation of laboratory test results is important. At some care levels, staff delivering the bulk of the care have not been trained to interpret laboratory findings. When a laboratory report identifies abnormal values, there may be no interpretation in the record that conveys whether the results are benign, alarming, or of any consequence at all. There may be a note in the physician's orders for a repeat test, but a retest order does not constitute an evaluation of the findings.

More frequently, there is neither an order for a retest nor other documentation that the abnormal results were not notable enough to warrant further testing. In most instances, the abnormal values are mentioned in the discharge summary, but providing the information at discharge does not help the clinicians while they are developing plans of care or delivering care. Nonmedical staff could greatly benefit from understanding the meaning of the laboratory results through the insertion of a physician's explanatory note. The note could be inserted into the sequential progress notes or within the documented history and physical.

EXAMPLES OF COMMUNICATION THROUGH USE OF EXPLANATORY NOTES

EXAMPLE The client has significantly elevated liver enzymes. They will probably decrease with continued sobriety. After 30 days of abstinence, he should be retested.

EXAMPLE There are many abnormal laboratory findings due to the eating disorder of the client. She has been placed on a special diet that will be closely monitored by nursing staff. Continuous retesting has been ordered. The laboratory findings are consistent with the fragile physical state of the client.

EXAMPLE The laboratory reports reveal several abnormal readings. Each is only slightly outside normal limits. No further testing will be conducted unless the physical condition of the client unexpectedly changes. The client is in good physical condition.

The final documentation challenge common to physical health care services is the need for an understandable evaluation of the findings or outcomes. This is particularly important at levels and in sites of care where the attending physician may not attend planning of care sessions, and communication occurs through documentation. What are recorded often are only raw data or diagnoses expressed in medical terminology. It is preferable that the information be communicated in less technical language so that those delivering the care, as well as the client, can better understand the nature of the findings.

EXAMPLES OF COMMUNICATION THROUGH NONTECHNICAL LANGUAGE

EXAMPLE A 15-year-old female is in good general physical health, but is 20 pounds overweight and suffers from severe acne and high cholesterol. She is being raised by a single parent who holds two jobs and cannot prepare meals for the family. As a result, the client creates her own menu, which she states is composed of "pizza, pop, and chocolate." Because of her weight, she is teased by her schoolmates. The teasing creates anxiety, which she handles by eating more. Her food choices increase her weight and cholesterol, establishing a vicious cycle. She should be seen by a dietitian as soon as it can be arranged.

EXAMPLE A 55-year-old male is relatively healthy despite 30 years of drinking. Laboratory results and the physical examination suggest some liver damage, but it is far less than might be expected given his history. It will probably clear with abstinence. The EKG suggests some minor abnormalities also. The recreation therapist should monitor his activities carefully until the repeat EKG is completed. He smokes heavily and shows early signs of some respiratory problems. It is recommended that part of the counseling focus on his need to quit smoking. Also recommended is a follow-up in six months to reevaluate the expected improvements resulting from abstinence.

Improving Physical Health Assessments and Care Documentation

The Introduction of this book states that a primary reason for the clinical/case record is communication. Communication requires that both the sender and the receiver of the information share an understanding of the language being used. The language of different professions is not always the same; therefore, each profession is obliged to ensure that when information is being communicated, it is understandable to those to whom it is being imparted. There is no difficulty with professionals within disciplines sharing information through the use of the "shorthand" common to that profession. However, when information is being conveyed to professionals outside one's discipline, it should be communicated in neutral language understandable to those receiving it, including the client. This concern is often most pronounced with the physical assessment.

It is common practice in 24-hour settings for a nonphysician to be the first staff person to assess a client's current and past physical problems. Frequently, the health screening/nursing assessment is completed as soon as possible upon onset of care or admission and before the physician's examination (as required by the standards or as indicated by the referral criteria).

The physician should comment on any salient information identified by other providers. This could be done in the documented history and physical or in a progress note. The documented review becomes particularly important when the health screening suggests the existence of a physical problem. In cases in which clients are referred to physicians outside the organization, it is very important that the staff's findings and concerns be communicated to the outside physician either verbally or in writing (such as by sending a copy of the health screening, and/or documenting the specific reasons for referral on a referral form).

Reviews of clinical/case records often reveal that physical problems detected by a nonphysician as reported by the client are not mentioned again in the written physical examination report completed by the physician. From a systems perspective, the "loop" is not closed. The absence of physician references to other providers' findings or complaints of the client make it unclear whether the identified issues were deemed unimportant or nonexistent or were merely overlooked by the physician. A brief entry in the clinical/case record by the physician would easily clarify the issue.

PHYSICIAN NOTES ON A NURSING ASSESSMENT

- Findings noted: Incorporated in history and physical.
- Findings noted: Recommendations can be found in dictated summary.
- No follow-up required.
- History of T13 noted. Arrange for chest x-ray.

Psychosocial Assessments

During the intake screening process, the provider conducts a preliminary screening of the emotional and mental status of the client to determine whether the site and level of care, treatment, or service being considered are appropriate. Major emphasis is placed on the lethality of the client (the degree of danger to self and/or others) and on whether the provider's level of care, treatment, and service affords adequate safety and security of the client. Because behavioral health care and social services are being sought, the professional conducting the intake should identify, at a minimum, the degree of behavioral health dysfunction the client is experiencing. A primary objective should be to determine the following:

- The severity of the condition of the client
- The least restrictive level of care, treatment, or service the client would be able to safely tolerate

The evaluation of a client's psychological functioning includes the following:

- Threat of harm to self or others
- The need for and intensity of supervision
- Barriers to processing information
- Potential neurological deficits, including cognitive deficits and disorientation
- Mood and affect
- Signs/symptoms of psychosis and/or other thought disorders

A more thorough evaluation of behavioral health and social issues is conducted after the decision to begin care, treatment, or service with the client is made. In crisis stabilization units and residential settings, the assessment is usually completed at admission and continuously expanded by the several clinicians and disciplines who carry out the assessment and care processes. Sections of the psychosocial assessment may be addressed within the admission assessment, continued by the physician during the physical examination, and repeated during the first meeting with the assigned counselor.

Providers are often subject to the demands of payers, regulatory agencies, and accrediting bodies that also specify the content of psychosocial assessments. Although the content may be very similar among payers, accreditors, and regulators, each may require unique refinements or use differences in language.

In all behavioral health care and social service settings, a psychiatric evaluation, mental health examination, psychological assessment, and evaluations of language, self-care, and visual-motor and cognitive functioning need to be conducted when indicated and may be performed by the appropriate staff of the organization or through a contractual agreement with other organizations or providers through referral.

In partial hospitalization, day care, intensive outpatient, adult day care, and outpatient settings, the assessment might not be fully completed within the first session because of time and program constraints.

Clients actively abusing alcohol or other drugs introduce special challenges to the psychosocial assessment. It may not be possible to accurately evaluate the behavioral health issues of clients who are under the influence of alcohol and/or drugs. The effects of the chemicals may cause the client to falsely appear mentally or emotionally dysfunctional, or they may mask serious problems. To protect against either possibility, the comprehensive psychosocial assessment of behavioral health problems for this population may be delayed until the client is physically free of the acute effects of alcohol or other drugs.

Cultural/Ethnic Assessments

In its assessment work, an organization should consider or evaluate the cultural, ethnic, or spiritual issues that impact planning of care. This is not necessarily a separate, formal assessment—it should be a component of the psychosocial assessment. Assessment standards require information on religion and spiritual orientation as well as information on family circumstances. This includes the configuration of the family group and social, ethnic, cultural, emotional, and health factors. The cultural/ethnic information is also required as a component of the assessment of the learning needs of the client and his or her family.

Despite the laudable advances in the understanding of mental illness, addictions, and the need for social supports within the United States, there remain those whose understanding is rooted in traditions and norms not generally shared by behavioral health care providers. This does not suggest that such beliefs are better or worse; they are merely different.

> Cultural background . . . has an important influence on many aspects of people's lives including their beliefs, behaviors, perceptions, emotions, language, religion, rituals, family structure, diet, dress, body image, concepts of space and time, and attitudes to illness, pain and other forms of misfortune—all of which may have important implications for health and health care.[3]

Issues related to culture and health care have become more significant in recent years as research is indicating disparities and/or inconsistencies in the delivery of care, treatment, and services for different populations. The Joint Commission and other organizations have recently made more information and resources available for organizations to keep in mind as they consider the care, treatment, and services that they provide in relation to the cultural backgrounds and sensitivities of the clients that they serve.[4]

It is important to evaluate a client's ethnic and cultural background to help determine what that client thinks and feels about the strengths, problems, needs, and desires he or she has. Clients often view their own strengths, problems, needs, and desires according to values and beliefs derived, in part, from their cultural backgrounds. A particular cultural or ethnic norm may reflect the view that behavioral health problems and social needs are retribution for moral lapses or are produced by malevolent spirits, or that addictions are willful behavior that can be simply and inexpensively relieved by maintaining a "Just say no" attitude. If a client was raised in an environment in which a certain behavior or condition was seen as demonic intercession, then that belief is bound to affect his or her recovery. If keeping emotions under tight control is a cultural virtue, then that client may find it difficult to share feelings or participate in psychodrama, which are required behaviors in some programs.

An evaluation of the ethnicity and cultural background of the client is more than a mere listing of his or her culture. It is not enough to state "client is Haitian," "client is Hispanic," or "client is African American." Those responses do not answer the following important questions:

- What—if anything—does coming from those backgrounds contribute to the current condition of the client?
- What are the cultural strengths and impediments that will affect the progress of the client?

Everyone is influenced by culture or multiple cultures. A more recent immigrant to the United States from China, for example, will be influenced by both Chinese and American culture. A second- or third-generation Chinese American will find themselves influenced by not only Chinese and American culture, but also by a kind of hybrid of both cultures born from the merging of the two. This is true for clients from all of the cultural and ethnic groups in the United States. Each has norms and beliefs about many issues: guilt, shame, unwed pregnancy, abortion, family, crime, goodness, evil, marriage, divorce, children, parents, the need for social services, alcoholism, mental illness, and personal responsibility, among many others.

In addition to influencing clients, cultural background or ethnicity affects the attitudes of family and friends and offers reliable clues about how the support system of the client can be relied on during recovery.

CULTURAL ASSESSMENTS

Assessment 1: Religious Irish-Catholic Woman with Divorce Guilt

This client was raised in an Irish Catholic family and is a first-generation American. She was married in a cathedral, with a bishop officiating the ceremony. Two years ago, she divorced her husband. The divorce repulsed her family, and her father still refuses to speak with her. She feels guilty and ashamed about her divorce and angry about her parents' abandonment. Intellectually, she thinks she did what was right. During childhood she was taught that a woman bore whatever burden was necessary to sustain a marriage, even an unhappy and abusive one. Until she is better able to forgive herself and/or confront her family about their lack of support, she will probably continue to be depressed.

Assessment 2: Puerto Rican Man with a Drinking Problem

This client was born in Puerto Rico. He thinks of himself as a virile male who should be able to "drink like a man." He does not want to appear dependent on females and may be initially resentful and resistant if assigned to a female addictions counselor. He embraces "macho" values and will find it difficult to accept that alcohol has overpowered him. All his friends drink and now ridicule him because he is getting help. He may have difficulty with Alcoholics Anonymous and with the concept of lifetime sobriety because it might mean having to change friends and values.

Assessment 3: White Homosexual Man with Family Problems

This client was raised in a white Anglo-Saxon Protestant home. His father had planned for him to take over the family accounting firm when he finished college. His parents and three siblings do not understand or accept his homosexuality. Given his upbringing, they cannot comprehend why he does not choose to behave like his heterosexual brothers. He expresses residual guilt about disappointing the family but is also angry because they will not accept him. He is particularly resentful that they refused to meet his companion, Bill, before he died from AIDS. The biological family attributes his problems and abandonment of their values to Bill's influence. Future biological family support will be difficult to generate. His current support group is composed of several close friends.

Spiritual Orientation Assessments

The term *spirituality* often defies precise definition. A spiritual assessment includes religious affiliation and such issues as the client's sense of life purpose, degree of isolation, and degree of alienation from others or from a higher power. In the interest of consistency and to improve the documentation processes, the provider may wish to establish a definition of spirituality to be used by the staff conducting spiritual assessments. While conducting spiritual assessments, staff would be expected to apply that definition.

Examples of assessment questions include the following:
- What are your values and beliefs?
- What motivates you?
- What is most important in your life?
- What are you most enthusiastic about?
- What or who is the love of your life?
- How much control do you feel you have over your life?

Figure 2-4 (*see* companion CD-ROM) contains a list of other potential spiritual assessment questions to ask clients. Examples of religious or spiritual assessments in which these questions have been applied appear below.

 Check the CD-ROM: A customizable version of Figure 2-4 is available for your organization's use on the companion CD-ROM.

RELIGIOUS/SPIRITUAL ASSESSMENTS

EXAMPLE Al is a self-professed atheist who appears to have a genuine love for his fellow man. He is optimistic about the future and hopes that he will be able to help other alcoholic atheists after his own sobriety is stabilized. He states that he cannot spend time thinking about a deity because it is too exhausting. He believes there is too much that needs to be done on earth among the living. Al's spiritual life appears to be adequate.

EXAMPLE Bob describes himself as a God-fearing man who is being punished for his life of excesses. He states that he has no religious affiliation, yet identifies his God as one of biblical justice—an eye for an eye. He expresses little hope for a future in paradise. Despite his strong beliefs in a higher power, Bob appears to have diminished spirituality, as demonstrated by his pessimism, self-condemnation, fear, and despair.

EXAMPLE Barbara is a lifelong Catholic who is trying to forgive herself for recent indiscretions. She has begun to make amends directly to those she has harmed. In some instances, her efforts have been accepted, but in other instances, they have been rejected. She continues anyway. She expresses hope and faith in the future and takes responsibility for the past. Her spiritual life is improving daily.

Improving Documentation in Psychosocial Assessments

Organizations should periodically review their psychosocial assessment tools to determine if they accurately identify the strengths, problems, or needs of their clients. For example, chemical dependency treatment programs often require clients to absorb a significant amount of education. The curriculum includes topics that require concentration and the ability to use abstract thought. One of the negative effects of most drugs and a major characteristic of alcohol abuse is the destruction or damage of brain cells; hence the cognitive ability of a client suffering from a substance-related disorder might be severely affected. A client who has difficulty remembering the way to the bathroom would likely receive little benefit from attending a required lecture on the topic of spirituality or family systems. A process that facilitates an evaluation of the client's cognitive functioning and ability to benefit from education would be clinically sensible before assigning a chair in the lecture hall.

The examples below show how a psychosocial summary might be written in such a way that both the client and the staff, regardless of discipline, would understand it. Because the examples demonstrate the use of clear language, they are brief and not intended to represent the content of a full psychosocial assessment. The psychosocial assessment is not limited to a description of the client's behavior. It also determines the ability of the client to benefit from the type and level of care, treatment, or service being offered.

UNDERSTANDABLE PSYCHOSOCIAL SUMMARIES (EXCERPTS)

EXAMPLE John's verbal responses to questions and his written answers suggest the possibility of short-term memory loss and other difficulties in processing information. It is likely that the problems are acute and will diminish or disappear after a period of abstinence. It is recommended that John be provided individual tutoring, using the computerized cognitive restructuring module. If his condition does not improve within seven days, a complete neurological examination should be scheduled.

EXAMPLE Susan's affect and mood suggest depression. She is frequently tearful and appears sad most of the time. She does not show any interest in interacting with other clients. She eats very little and often falls asleep during group therapy. She has not been placed on medication. It is recommended that a comprehensive psychiatric evaluation be completed before further changes are made to the plan of care.

Some providers use assessment forms that require the insertion of a comment after each psychosocial area. The form includes a list of important psychosocial areas, such as the following:

- Suicidal ideation
- Memory loss
- Hallucinations
- Panic attacks

- Delusions
- Prior care, treatment, or service

For many good reasons, providers fill in the blank spaces after each psychosocial area with the notation "denies." There is nothing wrong with this practice as long as there is some subsequent professional evaluation of the denials of the client. The client might be denying the items while chatting with an invisible companion about a suicide scheduled for later in the day. Or the client may deny that he is Napoleon but may now consider himself to be Julius Caesar. Documenting only what the client denies without some later evaluation renders the information incomplete. The purpose of any assessment is to evaluate the statements of the client, including his or her denials, which could be significant. It is the provider's responsibility to record the credibility of such denials. The following example reiterates the importance for further evaluation and documentation of a client's denials.

PROVIDERS' USE OF THE TERM *DENY*

EXAMPLE During the interview, Virginia denied being depressed or angry. Nonetheless, she frequently became tearful and had difficulty continuing the session. She acknowledged that she has difficulty sleeping at night and keeps thinking about the death of her spouse. She became animated during the discussion of her husband's sudden death and expressed her disappointment about his failure to take care of his health. Still, when asked whether she was angry about his leaving her abruptly, she denied it and said she had nothing but fond memories of him.

ANALYSIS OF ASSESSMENT DATA

Joint Commission standards require that organizations analyze or integrate data from various aspects of the screening/assessment and use the analysis to determine and prioritize the needs of the client. The standards focus on the process of analysis rather than on the documentation. However, the analysis is intended to consolidate the significant information gathered from the physical and psychosocial assessments of the client into a single evaluation. Therefore, providers do not have to develop a separate document called an Integrated Summary if another document or process blends the separate physical and psychosocial findings into a whole clinical portrait.

The purpose of the analysis is to ensure that when a portion of an assessment focuses on a single aspect of life (physical or psychosocial) of the client, the information is integrated with all the other aspects. When done effectively, the evaluation will allow identification and prioritization of the needs and strengths of the client.

This process may be performed during a team meeting, if that is the structure of the organization, and reflected in a progress note or meeting minutes. Other tools that can be used include a synthesized assessment and/or plan of care, discharge plan, problems/needs list, or practice guideline. A practice guideline describes the processes used to evaluate and treat a client having a specific diagnosis, condition, or symptom.

The primary provider for the client or an interdisciplinary team will implement a system for individualized assessment; care, treatment, or service; discharge; and education. Some providers use the psychiatric evaluation, psychological assessment, case history, or psychosocial history/summary as an analysis summary because, in their settings, these documents include the necessary information that captures the analysis of the assessment(s).

Although the analysis may contain some historical data and background, most of the content should be an analysis of that information. Some providers refer to the content as a *clinical* or *case formulation.* Others know it as a *clinical impression* or *impressions,* and yet others use the terms *conclusions* and/or *recommendations.* Whatever the label, the material should incorporate a complete assessment of the needs and strengths of the client.

Other Joint Commission standards (such as those addressing assessment and the continuum of care) that should be considered when developing a process to analyze and integrate significant information about the client include the following:

- Learning needs
- Coordination of care
- Referral, transfer, or discharge plan
- Discharge planning needs
- Plan of care reflecting the needs of the client

Providers are eminently qualified and ethically obligated to make judgments about assessment data; in fact, it is what they are paid to do. The purpose of collecting data about the client is to evaluate the client's expectations and need for care, treatment, or service; the kind of care, treatment, or service needed; the client's strengths, problems, and needs; and the targeted improvements. This evaluation or interpretation of data is critical to developing individualized care, treatment, or service plans and providing high-quality and safe care, treatment, or service.

Refer to the following examples of analyses of assessment data for further explanation.

WRITTEN ANALYSIS OF ASSESSMENT DATA

EXAMPLE Mary is a 45-year-old African American female who has reluctantly requested help from the behavioral health care service. Her life has become increasingly out of control during the past couple of years. She is unable to sleep more than four hours a night, resulting in chronic fatigue. She uses food to compensate for feelings of sadness or anxiety and is 40 pounds overweight. She suffers from loneliness and isolation.

Mary's husband is a successful lawyer who spends most of his time working. She resents her husband's success and his isolation from her, which she considers deliberate. She is also resentful about her sacrifices working at menial jobs to put him through law school while he now seems to have no time for her. She is unable to identify any positives about their relationship.

Mary's three children are busy with school activities, increasing her sense of isolation. She became agitated when discussing them, but suppressed any outward expression of hostility. Her anger was evident by the inflection and tone in her voice. Mary pursues leisure activities (for example, doing crosswords, reading, and watching television) that further isolate her and compound her loneliness, but she describes them as peaceful. She does not perceive that she has pulled away from others. She prefers to believe that others have abandoned her. The one positive thing in her life that she was able to identify is her job, but she has increasingly distanced herself from that through frequent absences. She has no close friends or emotional support system.

Mary appears to be in fair health but suffers from hypertension due in part to her weight. Despite a facade of calmness and passivity, she unwittingly showed anxiety by tapping her foot constantly, remaining very erect, and clenching her fist throughout the assessment process. She identified the church as her sole source of comfort but feels hypocritical about using the church as a vehicle to obtain forgiveness for sins committed as a teenager.

Mary is an intelligent and educated woman who lacks insight into her condition. She is not yet prepared to deal with her contributions to her situation. At one level, Mary thinks she deserves more out of life than she is realizing. At another, she is unable to identify personal resources she might tap into to attain a better life. She is passive and is relying on the behavioral health care service staff to provide her with a fail-safe recovery plan that she will merely have to put into place.

The first priority is to recommend a mental status evaluation. The second priority is to recommend a medication evaluation and schedule a nutritional assessment and a vocational assessment. The third priority is to engage her in therapy and determine the possibility of family support in treatment. Are family or marital issues appropriate for wife and husband? Finally, it is important to encourage her to reduce her isolation from friends and work, and to establish a structured plan for socialization with her family and friends.

EXAMPLE This is the second admission in the past six months for David, who is 15 years old. His parents, who are concerned about the recurrence of the behavior that prompted his first admission, referred him. He is again skipping school and sneaking out at night. His physical health remains good. All laboratory testing was within normal limits, and no unusual physical conditions were detected in the history and physical examinations. There is some evidence of dental needs, but they can be deferred until after discharge. David demonstrates distractible behavior. He has difficulty keeping the conversation focused on the topic. He was "squirmy" during the interview—he kept looking through the window to see what the clients outside were doing. His behavior was similar to that reported by his parents and by school officials. During the first admission, it was determined that he was experiencing attention-deficit/hyperactivity disorder (ADHD). He was placed on medication that stabilized his behavior. At the time of discharge, he was doing well in school both academically and behaviorally.

At the point of the original discharge, he and his parents were educated about the need for David to remain on the medication, but apparently none of them were convinced. Initially, David continued taking the medication as prescribed but began to miss doses and eventually stopped taking it altogether. He does not want to be seen by others (or by himself) as "a psycho." His parents do not seem able to set boundaries with David, and they are unable to ensure that he complies with the medication requirements. They seem to be passive clients who are looking for someone to "fix" their son.

David states that he hates his father and respects his mother, but he doesn't love her. He is an only child, appears to have been spoiled all his life, and responds negatively to limit setting. This, combined with the ADHD, creates problems for him in his relationships with adults.

He has been sneaking out late at night for a few hours and then returning home. It is possible that he is meeting with friends his parents describe as "druggies." David denies any drug use or abuse, but the issue should be watched and explored more fully. He states that he should not have to be subject to random drug screens. It is recommended that they be conducted despite his protests as long as there is parental approval. He also wants to smoke even though he has been advised of the no-smoking policy. This may be the first issue he challenges in relation to the program's limits.

David is of above-average intelligence and capable of being charming when he thinks it will get him what he wants. His family is supportive of the organization's efforts, although historically they have been ineffectual in following through with recommendations. Priorities are as follows: (1) stabilize him on medication, (2) return him successfully to school, and (3) begin family therapy to facilitate the implementation and enforcement of limit setting.

The remaining problems can be deferred until priorities 1 through 3 have been resolved.

In both of the above examples of assessment data analysis, the behavioral health care provider communicated the assets and needs of the client in clear terms so that problems/needs statements could be developed. An example of problems/needs statements for the client named Mary is seen in the box below. Problems/needs statements help to segue into the development of a more detailed problems/needs list for the client.

PROBLEMS/NEEDS STATEMENTS FOR MARY

Problem: The client is 40 pounds overweight.
Problem: The client sleeps only four hours per night.
Problem: The client is emotionally isolated from her husband, children, and friends.
Problem: The client's blood pressure is high at 160/100.

THE PROBLEMS/NEEDS LIST

The term *problems list* is used by some organizations, but terms such as *challenge list, areas to address, needs list,* and *problems/needs list* are used interchangeably. The last term, problems/needs list, might best capture the intent inasmuch as a need may well be different from a problem and yet require attention. For example, assume that Jim, an adolescent who has been treated successfully for ADHD with Ritalin, is admitted for care because of unrelated behavioral health issues. Jim needs to continue the medication while being treated for different behavioral health issues that prompted the admission. In this instance, the need is not a problem per se, but it would be included in the plan of care to ensure that the staff monitored Jim's compliance with the medication regimen. An example of an excerpt of a problems/needs list for Jim appears in the following box.

PROBLEMS/NEEDS LIST EXCERPT FOR JIM

Need: To continue with Ritalin as prescribed
Goal: To remain free of ADHD symptoms
Objective: Client will take Ritalin (10 mg) three times a day.
Intervention: Staff will observe client taking medication. Physician will review monthly for effectiveness.

As increasing numbers of providers participate in the continuum of care, a mechanism to track the emergence and status of the problems/needs of the client over a prolonged period becomes more important. Providers report that in an increasingly complicated world, the needs of the clients are becoming more complicated and that single or simple care issues are a rarity. The use of such a list affords greater certainty that each problem/need of the client will receive appropriate attention in a timely manner, either through direct care, treatment, or service; referral; or deferral. The problems/needs list serves as a tool to identify the active care issues, the issues that have been resolved, and those issues that have been referred to another provider or deferred for a later time.

There are many ways of using problems/needs lists, but they generally follow two broad processes:

✓ List each problem/need separately. The main advantage of itemizing the problems/needs is that when only one problem/need can be addressed at a time, there is a central site where unresolved ones are retained and can later be activated. *See* Figure 2-5, on the companion CD-ROM, for an example of an itemized problems/needs list for Mary.

✓ Group problems/needs into batches under a broad heading and then identify the behaviors that describe the broad heading as a subset (for example, family problems and depressed mood). *See* Figure 2-6 on the companion CD-ROM for a batched problems/needs list for Mary. The behaviors that define the headings are explicitly identified and follow the words "as evidenced by (AEB)."

 Check the CD-ROM: Customizable versions of Figures 2-5 and 2-6 are available for your organization's use on the companion CD-ROM.

THE NEED FOR PRECISE LANGUAGE

When clear language is used to communicate information in the clinical/case record, not only does it provide an accurate, well-described account of the care, treatment, and service experiences of the client being served, it also helps with other processes such as reimbursement, transfer to new levels of care, and discharge. It can also enhance the quality of multidisciplinary teamwork. Often, the different members of a team may learn initial information about a client from reviewing the clinical/case record. The more thorough and precise the language in the record is, the easier it will be to streamline and get the most out of any multidisciplinary meetings and teamwork.

Further, the use of precise language can enhance the quality of care, treatment, and services. The better the account of the assessment, plan of care, and progress notes for that client, the better the ability of the care providers to make any midstream adjustments or ensure that their work is meeting the potentially evolving or shifting needs of the client. Precise language can also help with client safety issues. If documentation points to an observation of a potential risky behavior that an initial assessment has discovered, care providers can put measures in place to help minimize a potential safety risk for the client.

In behavioral health care, *verbal communication* is usually clear, specific, and behaviorally oriented. Behavioral health care providers tend to be distinguished in the broader field of health care for their advanced and sophisticated interview and discussion techniques and can glean significant information from discussions with a client and in further evaluation and discussion with colleagues. This is not always the case with written communication, however, which can often be cloudy and imprecise. Behaviors that are detailed with clarity during discussions become camouflaged through the use of elaborate or "flowery" written terms.

Consider the following writing tips to assess and improve the precision of the language in your records:

✓ **Do a reverse assessment of the client based on the record only.** Imagine you have only the clinical/case record from which to glean information about a client. Pick a random record and do a blind review of the language in it. Review all of the documentation in the record and try to paint a picture of the client based only on what you have there. What does it tell you? Ask yourself: If you are a new provider working with this client, would you have enough information?

✓ **Identify your strongest writers and make them a resource.** From a review of your records, can you identify any particular staff members who have stronger writing skills in their documentation than others? Give them an opportunity to share with and mentor others in the organization. Ask them to share and document what they do when they prepare their documentation.

✓ **Ensure that you are up-to-date on abbreviations or terminology that should not be used.** Sometimes information in a clinical/case record can be unclear because of the use of misleading, confusing, or, even worse, unapproved abbreviations. Ensure that your staff are well educated on the abbreviations that should not be used, identify abbreviations or terminology that have caused confusion in the past, and prepare an internal list of "do not use" terms and abbreviations.

✓ **Keep the language simple.** While poetic or "flowery" language may have a significant and necessary role in the canon of literature, it is not suitable in a clinical/case record. Keeping in mind that the simplest and most straightforward language is probably the most effective for clinical/case record documentation, one rule of thumb should be that if the language is not clear enough to a person walking in off the street, it may need to be made clearer.

✓ **Provide additional training to staff.** Effective, concise, and precise writing is a skill that must be trained and practiced. Consider having documentation training workshops and share examples of what good documentation looks like versus what does not.

One writing technique many people use when they do not wish to be held accountable—or are not certain exactly what or how something should be written—is to be vague, but with sophistication and panache, using global, encompassing terms. This technique uses many qualifiers, adjectives and adverbs, obscure words, cryptic terms, and quotations from notable people. Documentation written with this technique may appear to be a masterpiece of eloquence. Upon closer scrutiny, however, the material is stilted. It lacks specificity about the behavioral nature of the problems/needs of the client. It sometimes has to be explained to other providers and translated for the client being served. The vocabulary and syntax, stunning as they may appear, are not useful. The writing is grand, but it unnecessarily obscures the issues that bring the client to care, treatment, or service.

EXAMPLE A client has admitted that she "shoplifts, lies, steals, and abuses drugs." The documentation states that the problem/need is "poor perceptual accuracy," and that the goal is "to improve the self-concept of the client." This has little to do with the behaviors of shoplifting, lying, stealing, or abusing drugs. The documentation would fail to conform to most organizations' policy or procedure requiring that all problems/needs statements and lists be written in behavioral, observable, and measurable terms. This documentation essentially states that the behavior is a product of the youth's poor and inaccurate perception of herself; she has a self-esteem problem. If staff were asked whether the client would have to demonstrate self-esteem before care would be completed, the answer would be "no." If staff were asked whether the client would have to stop shoplifting, stealing, lying, or abusing drugs, the response would be "yes." It was the behaviors that should have been documented as the targeted problems/needs, not poor perceptual accuracy.

Shoplifting, stealing, lying, and abusing drugs should be identified as problems (or needs) because of the following:
- They prompted the referral and admission.
- They were observable, thereby enabling them to be tracked.
- They were the behaviors discussed by staff during care, treatment, or service planning review sessions.
- Their elimination or reduction serves as a criterion for discharge.

Staff may think that such language is not professional enough, yet it is the very language they use when discussing the progress of the client. Staff rarely, if ever, discuss "poor perceptual accuracy."

This example illustrates the undue time and energy that can be spent attempting to be "professionally creative" or "professionally correct." It is an excellent example of how easy it would be to use plain language to replace pompous and vague terminology.

The following is a second example in which language disguises the issues that brought the client to care.

EXAMPLE The client is a 24-year-old male who has been referred because of acts of violence against family members. Problem number one on the plan of care was documented as "narcissistic injury." The term appears learned, complex, and challenging, but it doesn't communicate a clear picture of the problem or need. If a family member is asked why his or her relative was in care, it is unlikely that the response would be "he has a narcissistic injury."

What does the term mean? It is vague and immeasurable. If a staff member were to be asked why the client was admitted, he or she might promptly reply that whenever the client believed he was being judged or criticized, he abruptly hit people. He did not seek clarification; he did not count to 10 or turn the other cheek; he did not sort out his feelings; he punched people. If a asked about links between the behavior and the identified problem/need (narcissistic injury), the staff member would explain that, as a child, the client was constantly rebuked by his parents and made to feel inferior. Because they were his parents, he could not retaliate against them directly but would strike out at others. Therefore, he acted out anytime he felt he was being criticized or insulted. His violence was the result of childhood narcissistic injuries.

In both of these examples, staff had confused causation with behavior. Identifying causation is certainly important, but it does not guarantee elimination of that particular behavior. For instance, many people know why they feel depressed, but they are still depressed. In these examples, the clients were admitted not because of narcissistic injury or poor perceptual accuracy, or because their mothers and fathers lacked parenting skills—many people have parents like these, but they resist punching perceived adversaries. These two clients were admitted because of behaviors that were problematic for them and others.

Another challenge is how to individualize the portraits of clients who have similar backgrounds and similar problems/needs. For example, the presenting problems/needs of clients with alcohol and drug issues often appear to be similar. Most have demonstrable problems/needs in one or more of the areas identified in the following box, which shows examples of incomplete problems/needs statements. If the problems/needs are documented without elaboration, as they are in these examples, then they are not serious enough to justify admission to any level of care, treatment, or service. Even some abstainers have such problems/needs. Other people, who do drink, have similar difficulties, but in their cases the problems/needs are unrelated to their drinking. There are also many people who possess the same traits but who are not candidates for care, treatment, or service. And yet others—who drink and should be receiving care, treatment, or service—manifest behavioral problems/needs different from those in these examples. What is needed are more precise definitions of the problems/needs and/or individualization of them.

EXAMPLES OF INCOMPLETE WRITTEN PROBLEMS/NEEDS STATEMENTS

- Lacks understanding of the disease concept
- Job problems
- Denial
- Legal problems
- Family problems
- Low self-esteem

To improve documentation, it is more effective to identify the specific difficulty a particular client might have within any of the given categories. For example, "lacks understanding of the disease concept" does not define exactly how it applies to Client A, B, or C.

- What specifically does the client not understand? The concept of disease? The concept of addiction as a disease? All of the concept or part of the concept?
- Is the problem the client's lack of understanding or inability to apply the concept?

Clients may understand the disease concept very well but not have the slightest idea how to alleviate their dependency. There are clients who could teach the disease concept as adeptly as the staff because they have heard it so many times during multiple treatment admissions, yet they cannot get their chemical dependencies or their lives under control.

In one addiction program in which "lacks understanding of the disease concept" was listed on every plan of care, the primary counselor was asked what specifically Client A did not understand. The answer was: "He believes that if he drinks only on weekends and drinks only beer, he will have no problems. Based on his history of weekend binges and Saturday night arrests for domestic violence, it is my clinical judgment that he is not safe drinking anything, anytime." The counselor had identified a specific error in the logic, thinking, recall, and belief systems of the client. There was specificity about what the client did not understand in relation to the disease concept.

In another example, the plan of care for Client B identified the same issue as for Client A: "Lacks understanding of the disease concept." The primary counselor was asked what it was about the disease concept that this client did not understand. The response was that the client agreed that he couldn't drink alcohol at all, but saw nothing wrong with sharing a couple of marijuana joints after work with his wife and teenage children. The counselor accurately verbalized the problem of the client but used the generic problem in nonspecific writing. Table 2-1, page 44, demonstrates how nonspecific terms can be converted into more behavioral and individualized language.

Table 2-1

Converting Nonspecific Terms into Behavioral and Individualized Language

Client A
Nonspecific: Lacks understanding of the effects of alcohol abuse.
Clarifier: As shown by the following: Client thinks that by switching from hard alcohol to beer he will have no further difficulty. Client sees no relationship between his four weekend arrests for domestic violence and drinking alcohol.

Client B
Nonspecific: Family problems
Clarifier: As demonstrated by the following: Client considers smoking marijuana with his wife and children to be a healthy family experience. Client does not understand how smoking marijuana might become a dependency, like that of alcohol.

The addition of the clarifying statements demonstrates the difference between the clients and represents the issues that were genuinely receiving counselor attention. The problems/needs statements become utilitarian. The examples also reflect how to batch clarifying behaviors under a broad descriptor.

It should be further noted that the terms *as demonstrated by* and *as shown by* were inserted below the descriptor. Other phrases commonly used are *as evidenced by* and *as manifested by*. The practical purpose for the insertion of the three words is that it requires the person writing the material to include observable activities of the client. It is the observable activity of the client that prompts care, treatment, or service and reflects progress. Such activity (or behavior) comprises the content of staff discussions about the client. When it is documented throughout the process of care, there is a direct relationship between the clinical/case record and the care, treatment, or service that is being delivered.

EXAMPLE "Impaired social skills" was the documented primary problem for a client who had been a resident in a state psychiatric facility for 30 years and had been released as part of a community-based project. During planning of care sessions, the case manager specifically identified the problematic issues of the client as his refusal to take baths regularly and his refusal to change his clothes at all. The group home manager, the staff, and his housemates were eager for the client to change his habits or change his address.

During planning sessions, the case manager and other staff spoke very directly about the behavior of the client and their hopes for teaching him improved hygiene. They focused on his resistance to take baths and change his clothes. When asked why the specific problems that the staff had identified and were actively addressing were not documented, the case manager stated that somehow not taking baths and not changing clothes did not sound sufficiently sophisticated.

The case manger was correct in stating that the behaviors of the client were not clinically complex. They were, however, very important to the client. Moreover, the staff members were working to help the client acquire skills that would enable him to live more congenially among his housemates and to remain in the community.

In the above example, staff had identified a very serious problem—impaired social skills—but had not individualized it, even though they were expending enormous energy trying to remedy specific problem behaviors. It would have been much easier and far more efficient to merely put in writing what they were addressing. Table 2-2, below, illustrates how it could have appeared. When problem statements are documented as clearly as in Table 2-2, the treatment objectives almost write themselves. The major difficulty in developing effective plans of care is the failure to document problems/needs in terms of specific behaviors. The more specifically a problem is documented, the simpler it is to write care objectives and the easier it is for the client to identify and understand them.

Clients do not enter care, treatment, or service because of lofty or sublime issues. The reason for admission is usually unpleasant or unattractive behavior that harms the client and/or others, or prevents the client from adequately functioning in daily life. Such behaviors or conditions as hallucinations, delusions, suicide, self-loathing, incest, anorexia, and paranoia should not be disguised.

There are other catch-all, imprecise problems/needs statements in clinical/case records that could also be improved by adding some clarifiers. One, in particular, appears among all age groups, in all settings, and at all levels of care. It is an illusory phrase, perhaps applicable to every person at one point or another during a lifetime: "low (or poor or diminished) self-esteem." If behavioral health care records are valid indicators, there is a nationwide epidemic of low self-esteem. This phrase is used to defend the need for care for sexual "addiction" and frigidity, for overworking and indolence, for overeating and anorexia, and for personal isolation and emotional confusion.

Low self-esteem can be a very serious problem and can be closely associated with behavioral health problems. When entering it in the record, the challenge is to provide specific behavioral descriptions of how Client A's low self-esteem is distinguished from that of Client B. If the assessments of Client A and Client B state that each is suffering from low self-esteem, without further clarifying information, there is no way to differentiate the two.

Table 2-2

Making Problems/Needs Statements More Specific

Nonspecific: Impaired social skills
Clarifier: As manifested by the following:
   a. Client refuses to bathe.
   b. Client refuses to change clothes.

Nonspecific: Poor personal hygiene
Clarifier: As evidenced by the following:
   a. Client refuses to bathe and has not had a bath in one month.
   b. Client refuses to change his clothes and has worn the same clothing for six months.

> **EXAMPLE** A client named Jane enters treatment. She appears in ill-fitting clothing, has not combed her hair, makes numerous critical comments about herself, and remains aloof from other clients. It might be the staff's conclusion that she is experiencing low self-esteem, and that problem is placed on the problems/needs statement or list and plan of care.
>
> Now assume a second client named Anne is admitted. Anne never interacts with the staff or other clients unless she is dressed immaculately. She changes clothes several times a day, particularly if a crease or a spot of dirt appears on any garment, and she never has a hair out of place. She is never alone and seeks the companionship of peers or staff unceasingly. Anne freely shares her accomplishments in the arts and sciences with all who will listen. We witness the same staff, same program, same identified problem: low self-esteem. But Anne's behavior is the opposite of Jane's behavior.
>
> If we were to sit in on a meeting to review Jane's progress, the staff would not be apt to ask, "How is Jane's self-esteem?" They would be much more prone to comment on whether or not she had started mingling with other clients, combing her hair, washing and pressing her clothing, and saying positive things about herself. How else could progress ever be measured? When discussing Anne, the staff would be commenting on whether she had stopped changing clothes incessantly, was more comfortable with solitude, and had reduced the amount of talking about her talents.

The importance of behavioral descriptors to differentiate clients cannot be overemphasized. Table 2-3, below, demonstrates problems/needs statements for Jane and Anne.

There is no clinical or administrative reason why encompassing descriptive terms such as *low self-esteem, denial,* or *poor impulse control* should not be used if they are further defined in terms of the behaviors of the client.

In a final example, assume that a case manager has completed an assessment of a youth and prioritizes poor impulse control as the problem to be first addressed in care, treatment, or service. Poor impulse control is a characteristic of most youths—and many adults—both in and out of care, treat-

---

Table 2-3

Problems/Needs Statements

Jane
Problem Number 1
Nonspecific: Low self-esteem
Clarifier: As demonstrated by isolation from other clients, poor hygiene, rumpled clothing, and frequent negative comments about self

Anne
Problem Number 1
Nonspecific: Low self-esteem
Clarifier: As shown by the need for constant companionship, frequent preening, combing hair, immaculate dress (changes clothes at least four times a day), and continuous boasting about accomplishments

---

Table 2-4

Use of Behavioral Descriptors

Jared
Problem Number 1
Nonspecific: Poor impulse control
Clarifier: As demonstrated by using physical force with peers when frustrated, leaving the classroom without permission, and stealing property from others

---

ment, or service. If only the three words *poor impulse control* are recorded on the problems/needs statement or list or plan of care, then very little has been communicated to other staff members, to the client, or to payers about the specific characteristics of that client. However, if poor impulse control is modified by the addition of behavioral descriptors, then meaningful communication will have occurred. The example in Table 2-4, above, demonstrates the use of behavioral descriptors for a client named Jared.

When discussing Jared, the staff will probably focus on whether he is still striking others when frustrated, leaving the classroom, stealing, or demonstrating any other behaviors that reflect poor impulse control. It is unlikely that the staff will be asked: "How is Jared's poor impulse control coming along?"

SUMMARY

Assessment includes both the collection of data and its evaluation or interpretation. Such tasks as taking a history, conducting an examination, or testing the client are important functions, but if they do not result in a written evaluation of the results, then only half of the assessment process has been completed. It is not enough to merely have a written evaluation—that evaluation should be precisely written so that the record paints a thorough and accurate picture of the client, the plan of care laid out for him or her, and the progress that he or she is making.

Clients enter care, treatment, or service because of problems or needs related to their behavior. Problems/needs statements or lists should therefore describe each problem or need in observable, behavioral, and (whenever possible) measurable terms. Only in that way can progress be tracked. It is the behaviors of the clients that get them into care, treatment, or service, and it is their new behaviors that get them out of care, treatment, or service.

Assessment is care; it is not an event to be rapidly completed so that care can begin. The quality of the assessment process governs care outcomes.

Financial resources for health care, particularly those in behavioral health care and social services, remain limited. There has never been more urgency for behavioral health care and social service providers to champion the rights of the clients they serve to receive adequate care. Advocacy will require outcome data, and the clinical/case record will have to be relied upon as a rich source of information.

REFERENCES

1. Bodek H.: *Standards for Clinical Documentation and Recordkeeping.* New York State Society for Clinical Social Work. http://www.clinicalsw.org/basic_standards.html (accessed Sep. 15, 2007).

2. Epstein M.H., Sharma J.M.: *Behavioral and Emotional Rating Scale: A Strength-Based Approach to Assessment.* Austin, TX: Pro-Ed, 1998.

3. Helman C.G.: *Culture, Health, and Illness,* 3rd ed. Boston: Butterworth-Heinemann Ltd., 1994.

4. The Joint Commission: *Hospitals, Language, and Culture: A Snapshot of the Nation, Compiled List of Resources.* 2007. http://www.jointcommission.org/PatientSafety/HLC/compiled_list.htm (accessed Sep. 16, 2007).

Section 3

THE PROCESS AND STRUCTURE OF PLANNING OF CARE

ASPECTS OF THE PLANNING OF CARE PROCESS

A plan of care (or a treatment or service plan) is exactly what the term implies: a blueprint, a design, and a projected strategy. Like any blueprint, the plan of care is susceptible to frequent revision in response to changes in the needs of the client. Sidebar 3-1, page 50, identifies key terms that are used in this discussion of plans of care.

Because the primary intent of the plan of care is to facilitate behavioral improvement, it is reasonable to expect such change and to modify the plan whenever behavioral objectives have been attained. The plan is intended to be a guide to care based on the information available at the time that it is developed and each time it is revised. As new information is gathered, the plan is subject to revision. Goals and objectives may be modified. Interventions may be increased, decreased, changed, or discontinued; target dates for achievement may be altered. The plan of care should be conceptualized as a continuous sequence of mini-plans that result in incremental progress from the time of entry to discharge or transfer.

In some situations, such as plans of care for persons with developmental disabilities, progress may not be "discharge or transfer." And for some aspects of emotional disorders the goal may not be incremental progress. Establishing a goal to maintain the current level of functioning and/or decrease the rate of loss of function may be the goal in such cases. Progress may be sought to a given level and then maintained at that level. If this is the realistic goal, stating it accordingly is acceptable.

Revisions, additions, deletions, or modifications of a plan should not be considered undesirable consequences of a flawed process. Rather, plan of care revisions demonstrate that the process is working as it should. Figure 3-1, page 51, is an example of the planning of care process.

Effective plans of care generate demonstrable improvement of the client, which should prompt new or revised care objectives and interventions. If a plan of care remains unchanged, particularly for a client who remains within a continuum of care for a prolonged period, the following assumptions might be made:

- There has been no demonstrable improvement or regression of the client.
- The documented plan is so vaguely written that change in the client's behavior is not observable.
- Documenting the plan of care was perceived as an "event," and the staff now considers that event to be history.
- No one has looked at the plan lately.
- The client has eloped and is unavailable for monitoring.

Sidebar 3-1

Key Planning of Care Terms

Continuing plan of care: A documented plan of action developed before discharge or transfer to another level of care. The purpose of the plan is to assist the client in sustaining the progress that has been achieved through linkage with supportive resources located in the environment to which the client is being returned. The continuing plan of care is sometimes included within a discharge summary or is recorded in a separate planning document.

Criteria for discharge: Statements that guide staff in knowing when the client is ready for discharge or transfer. These criteria might be one and the same as clearly written objectives, or they can be separate statements included in the plan of care. Discharge criteria should be consistent with or may be guided by any formal placement criteria.

Goals: Broad and encompassing statements of desirable behavioral change that a client should achieve to reflect maximum or optimal care outcome. (Some providers use the term *long-term goals.*) A logical and specific relationship should exist between each goal and each identified active problem/need.

Interventions: Planned procedures designed by the staff to bring about the behavioral changes identified in the care objectives. Interventions include any assignments given to the client. The frequency of interventions and the name of the provider (whenever possible) or the discipline responsible for carrying out the intervention should be documented. Interventions may also be identified as *strategies, methods, steps,* or *modalities.*

Objectives: Statements of desirable, observable, and measurable behavioral change that demonstrate the achievement of the steps necessary to meet the goal. For instance, in problem-oriented plans of care, the objectives reflect the measurable behavioral changes that demonstrate the elimination or significant reduction of the identified client problems. In need-oriented plans of care, the objectives reflect the measurable behavioral changes that demonstrate the gaining of knowledge or insight, the planning/practicing/gaining of skills, or the application of skills to particular situations. Objectives are directly related to the goals and the identified active problems/needs. The term *short-term goals* is sometimes used instead of *objectives.* In rare instances, other terms, such as *challenges,* are used. Each objective should include an anticipated time frame of achievement.

Progress notes: Sequential narratives that depict the progress of the client in relation to the plan of care. They may also be used to record other significant events.

Care (or treatment or service) plan: A plan, based on data gathered during the assessment, that identifies the care, treatment, or service needs of the client, lists the strategy for providing services to meet those needs, documents care goals and objectives, and outlines the criteria for terminating specified interventions. The format of the plan in some organizations may be guided by protocols, practice guidelines, or a combination of several methods.

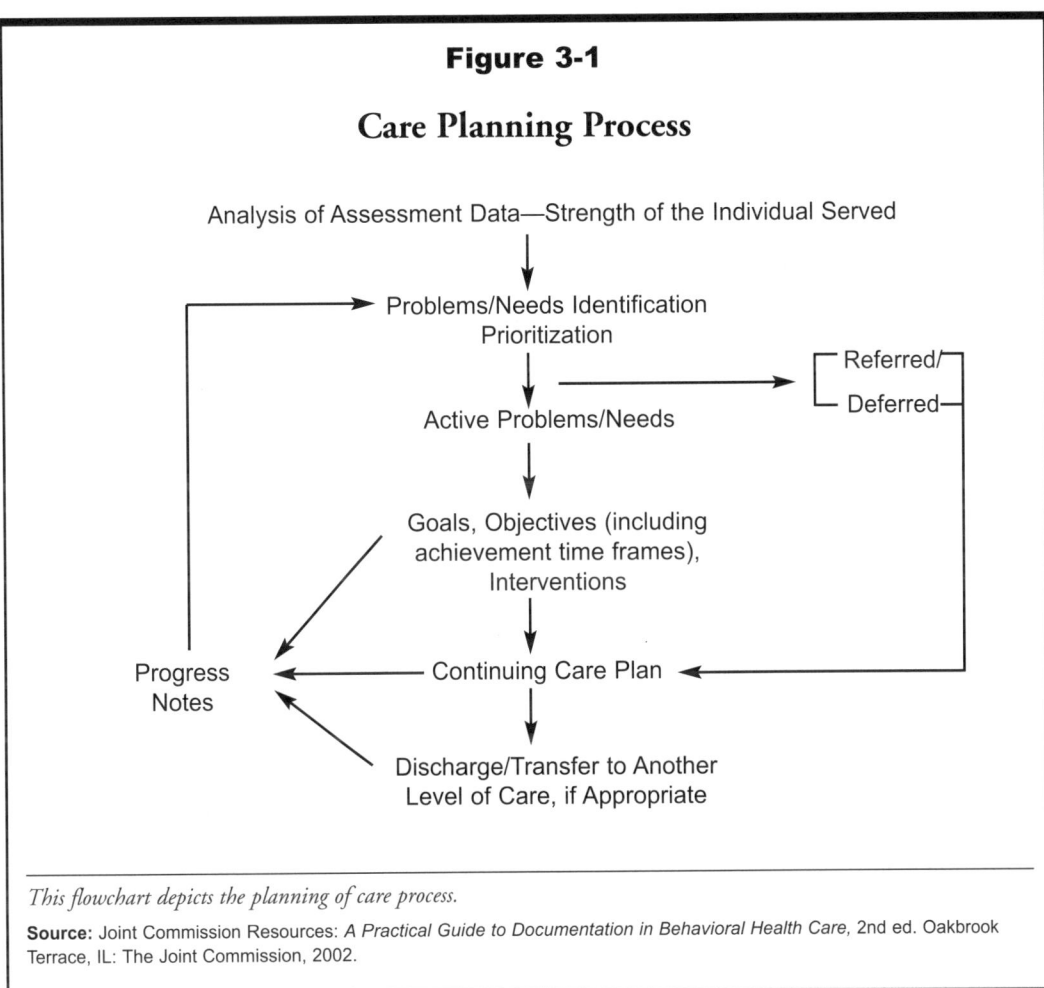

Figure 3-1

Care Planning Process

This flowchart depicts the planning of care process.

Source: Joint Commission Resources: *A Practical Guide to Documentation in Behavioral Health Care,* 2nd ed. Oakbrook Terrace, IL: The Joint Commission, 2002.

Perhaps these are unfair assumptions, but it may not be difficult, during random reviews of clinical/case records, to locate plans of care in mostly pristine states, even though the client has been in care for an extended period of time. Sidebar 3-2, page 52, identifies the traits that characterize effective and practical plans of care.

A first step in the planning of care process is to consider the stated goals of the client (and their families, as appropriate) and reevaluate the needs of the client in the problems/needs list or analysis of assessment data to determine that the problems/needs are clearly written, behaviorally defined, and appropriately prioritized. As discussed in Section 2, it is critical to identify the needs of the client in observable, behavioral terms. *Behavioral terms* have been defined as those thoughts, actions, or feelings that reflect the impairments of the client or prevent or interfere with the skills of the client and support requirements for living, learning, and work/educational activities. When the problems/needs statements are well written, the development of care goals and objectives is a simpler process. If problems/needs statements are vague and unclear, the development of observable care goals and objectives is laborious or impossible (*see* the example in the box on page 52 and the discussion that follows it). Staff attitudes about the wastefulness of documentation then become self-reinforcing.

Sidebar 3-2

Traits of Effective Care, Treatment, or Service Plans

- Effective plans are flexible. They are capable of being changed.
- Effective plans are realistic. Objectives are achievable, observable, and measurable.
- Effective plans are simple. Clients, family, and staff can understand them. They are written in plain language.
- Effective plans are useful. They provide measurable indicators of progress.
- Effective plans reflect and identify the client's condition (behaviors) that support care services.
- Effective plans identify presenting conditions, problems, or needs that will be addressed during care, treatment, or service; those that will be referred to other providers; and those that will be deferred to another time.
- Effective plans identify why the care, treatment, or service is necessary; why the setting is appropriate; and why alternative interventions are not considered appropriate.
- Effective plans include the changes that are anticipated for the client (goals and objectives) and their anticipated achievement time frames (target dates).
- Effective plans clearly identify the type and frequency of interventions. Staff know what they should do (methods, actions, and approaches) and how often they should do it.
- Effective plans identify the condition of the client upon completion of care, treatment, or service (outcome).
- Effective plans identify the plan to address the ongoing needs of the client (transfer, discharge, or aftercare plan).
- Effective plans support the need of the client for the level and length of care, treatment, or service being provided.
- Effective plans reflect what changes in the client would prompt a discharge/transfer.
- Effective plans facilitate interdisciplinary collaboration if a multidisciplinary team is providing care, treatment, or service.

VAGUE PROBLEMS/NEEDS STATEMENT

EXAMPLE Fred is a 45-year-old male who was admitted to care because of another episode of unusual and uncontrollable behavior. He had successfully made arrangements to acquire a hotel in Florida despite having no money. He telephoned people whom he had not seen in many years to interest them in investing or staying in his new hotel. He also began writing a screenplay—including a musical score—and intended to complete it in three days. He had gone without sleep for 60 hours and had not eaten in 2 days. The documentation for Fred's case was incomplete and unclear, containing only a provisional diagnosis of a bipolar disorder. The psychiatrist prescribed medication that tempered some of the hyperactive and hypervigilant behaviors, but insufficient time had passed for the behaviors to be brought under full control. Fred is now trying to persuade other clients to invest in his hotel or in the movie he wants to produce and direct. He is also resistant to taking medication.

As Fred's case demonstrates, if the condition alone (for example, depression, attention-deficit/hyperactivity disorder, or oppositional defiant disorder) is documented as a problem or need on the plan of care, it is difficult to establish goals and objectives. Sometimes conditions are documented as problems of the client. Standing alone, conditions (or diagnoses) are incorrectly expressed as problems/needs statements because they lack specificity and individualization. If the term "*manic behavior*" was recorded as the problem statement, there might be a slightly better understanding of the problem, but specificity would still be lacking. It would continue to be unclear how Fred's manic behavior differentiated him from every other client who was experiencing the same problem. But if Fred's specific behaviors were added to the problems/needs statement, the ability to document observable goals and objectives would be enhanced. Examples of how a condition or broad problems/needs statement might be used on a plan of care are shown in Figures 3-2 and 3-3, pages 54–55. The figures contain different plan of care formats to demonstrate that it is the *content* of documents rather than their format that reflects the quality of the process.

> **Check the CD-ROM:** A customizable version of Figures 3-2 and 3-3 are available for your organization's use on the companion CD-ROM.

Note that in Figure 3-2 a single plan of care form is used for each identified problem/need. Additional problems/needs would be placed on separate forms. A diagnosis was used as the active problem/need, but it was more precisely defined and individualized by the addition of specific individual behaviors. The goal has a logical relationship to the problem/need. The objectives are observable and reflect either elimination or a significant reduction of the behaviors that prompted care. The interventions and their frequency are cited, and the identity of the staff person or discipline responsible for carrying out the interventions is specifically noted. The objectives also serve as criteria for discharge/transfer. Anyone could use the plan to track the progress of the client.

Figure 3-3 uses a broad descriptor of the problems/needs of the client rather than a diagnosis. It includes clarifiers that precisely identify the behaviors defining that broad term. As can be observed, the behaviors are described somewhat differently from those in Figure 3-2, but the essential nature of the behaviors is very much the same. The differences are due to how each provider perceived the nature of the issues. The form in Figure 3-3 allows for the listing of sequential problems/needs.

A simple test can be used to evaluate the quality of documentation. Providers can pose the questions listed in Figure 3-4, page 56, to evaluate their documentation skills. Assuming that the answer to each of the questions in Figure 3-4 is "yes" and that the problems are clear in everyone's mind (including the client's), the next step would be to establish the goals and objectives for each problem.

> **Check the CD-ROM:** A customizable version of Figure 3-4 is available for your organization's use on the companion CD-ROM.

A goal is the end point of care in relation to the identified problem/need. It is a condition that will be reached only after a prolonged period. Goals are those improved conditions of the client that broadly reflect the optimal, acceptable elimination of a problem. Sidebar 3-3, page 56, provides some examples of goal statements.

Objectives are those desired behaviors that show that the problem(s) of the client is either gone or sufficiently alleviated to permit discharge or a transfer to another level of care (with the exception of opioid treatment programs). The problem/need may be a thought, an emotion, or an action that ultimately creates a problem for the client and/or others. Table 3-1, page 57, identifies relatively vague care objectives and illustrates how they can be clarified.

Figure 3-2

Interdisciplinary Care Plan
(Addressing a Single Problem/Need)

Date Identified: 1/20/XX

Identified by: WM, PhD

No.: 1   **Problem:** Bipolar disorder hypomanic episode as demonstrated by:
a) Sleeplessness (for $2\frac{1}{2}$ days straight)
b) Grandiosity (purchased hotel without having money, writing screenplay and musical score)
c) Pressured speech

Goal: To reduce/eliminate hypomanic behavior.

Date	Problem Number	Objectives/Time Frame (desired behavioral change)	Intervention/Frequency (care provided to achieve objective: what and how often)	Staff/ Discipline	Projected Achievement Date
1/20/XX	1a	Individual served will sleep 8 hours without interruption.*	1a Relaxation exercises-daily Lithium-daily	Nursing Nursing	1/22/XX*
	1b	Individual served will postpone preparation of movie script and musical score.*	1b Individual psychotherapy-daily Group therapy-daily	C. Domille, PhD. O. Stone, MSW	1/27/XX*
	1c	Individual served will discontinue phone calls to friends around country. Will request to make only two calls per day.*	1c Individual psychotherapy-daily Group therapy-daily	C. Domille, PhD. O. Stone, MSW	1/28/XX*

* Criteria for discharge _____   Date _____
Individual Served

_____   Date _____
Case Manager

This figure shows a single plan of care form for each identified problem/need.

Source: Joint Commission Resources: *A Practical Guide to Documentation in Behavioral Health Care,* 2nd ed. Oakbrook Terrace, IL: The Joint Commission, 2002.

Figure 3-3

Interdisciplinary Care Plan
(Addressing Multiple Problems/Needs)

Problem Number _____ Meeting Date: 1/20/XX

1   **Updated or New Problem:**
           Hypomanic behavior as manifested by:
           1a)   Sleeplessness for 2½ days
           1b)   Inflated self–esteem (writing screenplay/musical score)
           1c)   Pressured speech (lost voice today)

           Goal:
           To bring hypomanic behavior under control.

           Objectives:
           1a)   Will sleep 8 hours each night for three consecutive nights.
           1b)   Will acknowledge that writing screenplay and score in three days is
                  unrealistic.
           1c)   Will stop calling friends and will spend fewer than 15
                  minutes on the phone each day.

           Staff Plan of Care (including responsibility):
           1a)   Recreation staff will teach relaxation techniques. Physician will prescribe
                  medication and staff will administer it.
           1b/c) Psychologist will provide individual therapy daily. Social worker will
                  conduct group therapy daily.

           Critical for Discharge: Achievement of objectives.

Anticipated Date of Achievement: 1a) 1/22/XX   1b) 1/27/XX   1c) 1/27/XX
Staff Signature/Date: _____

Problem Number _____ Meeting Date:1/20/XX

2   **Updated or New Problem:**
           Individual resistant to medication

           Goal:
           To stabilize medication intake of the individual served.

           Objective:
           Individual served will take medication as prescribed for three consecutive days
           without staff coercion.

           Staff Plan of Care (including responsibility):
           • Educate individual served about purpose and need for medication.
           • Nursing staff will provide daily until individual assumes responsibility.
           • Psychologist will also provide motivational strategies during daily individual
             sessions.

Anticipated Date of Achievement: 1/30/XX
Staff Signature/Date: _____
Signature of Physician: _____
Signature of Individual Served: _____
Staff Present: _____

This figure uses a broad description of the problems/needs of the individual served.

Source: Joint Commission Resources: *A Practical Guide to Documentation in Behavioral Health Care,* 2nd ed. Oakbrook
Terrace, IL: The Joint Commission, 2002.

Figure 3-4

Questions to Evaluate the Quality of Documentation

☐ Do the problems/needs statements describe the behavior of the client in observable terms?

☐ Can staff see (or hear) the behaviors identified as problems or needs so that behavioral change will be detectable when it occurs?

☐ Are the problems/needs statements unique to this client, or could they apply to numerous other clients?

☐ Is it clear what the client has to do, say, learn, apply, and/or demonstrate that would prompt discharge/transfer?

☐ Are the objectives written in a manner that provides a basis for assessing progress during care reviews?

☐ If the problems/needs statements by themselves were read to the providers, and the name of the client was withheld, would the providers be able to identify the client?

This figure offers questions to aid in evaluating documentation.

Sidebar 3-3

Goal Statements

- To obtain employment
- To improve family life
- To achieve sobriety
- To complete school
- To improve physical health

By examining the objectives in Table 3-1, page 57, it should be simple to deduce the nature of the problem, even if the problems/needs statement has not been read. One way to think about the relationship between problems/needs statements and care objectives is to compare it with the use of a compass in order to get away from an unpleasant environment. The destination (that is, care objective) should be 180 degrees (or as close as possible to 180 degrees) from the unpleasant environment (problem/need).

Table 3-1

Rewritten Care Objectives

Imprecise: John will be free of psychotic symptoms.
Explicit: John will be free of hallucinations and delusions for 72 consecutive hours.

Imprecise: Mary will improve her sleeping habits.
Explicit: Mary will sleep eight hours without interruption.

Imprecise: Barbara will overcome her weight problem.
Explicit: Barbara will lose five pounds by 1/19/XX.

Imprecise: Fred will reduce his manic behavior.
Explicit: Fred will make only two five-minute phone calls a day—one to his spouse and one to his parents.

Imprecise: Bill will improve his hygiene.
Explicit: Bill will take a shower each morning and put on clean clothing before leaving home.

Imprecise: Charlie will accept his alcoholism.
Explicit: Charlie will voluntarily acknowledge that he is unable to stop drinking once he starts, regardless of what alcoholic beverage he is consuming.

Consider an example involving a youth, Bob, who has been referred for care. The evaluation shows that Bob prefers to blame his negative behavior on others and avoid assuming personal responsibility. The case manager documents the problem as follows:

Problem 1: Bob does not assume responsibility for his actions as evidenced by his statement that he has never gotten into trouble on his own. He attributes his problems at home, at school, and with the law to hanging out with the wrong companions and taking the blame for their actions.

Goal: To take more personal responsibility

Care Objective: By week 4, Bob will acknowledge five episodes in which he got into trouble due to his own behavior either at school, with the police, or when he was alone.

If anyone were to read the objective without having read the problem, he or she would easily deduce that Bob has difficulty identifying his own contributions to getting into trouble. There is congruence between the central themes in the goal, the problem statement, and the care objective. In this instance, the objective is 180 degrees from the problem; it represents an erasure of the problem. In many instances, a 100% erasure of the problem may not be feasible. In those situations, the staff and clients may be satisfied with only 160 or 140 degrees of improvement because it serves as a criterion for transfer to a less intense/less restrictive level of care, treatment, or service. As a client moves from level to level, there will be incremental behavioral improvement, so eventually the behavior comes close to being totally eradicated.

There is a simple way for providers to check the strength and validity of the objectives that have been written. First, they should read the objective(s) and then read the problems/needs statement. If the two are logically linked, the objective should eliminate the identified problem/need, or at least begin to reduce its negative impact to a level that permits the client to function.

Providers continuously monitor the conditions that created the need for the care of a client and whether or not these conditions are disappearing. If an objective does not reflect a removal or significant reduction of the identified problem, change in behavior, or attainment of a new skill, the cause may be a poorly defined problems/needs statement. On the other hand, the objective may be valid but related to a different problem/need. Alternatively, the objective may not be written well. In some situations, providers are often far more proficient in identifying the changes a client should be striving for than they are in documenting problems/needs. If this is the case, providers will find that by writing the objective (that is, the desired behavioral changes) first, the problem/need writes itself. They can then "back into" the problem statement.

After the problems/needs have been defined and prioritized and the improved behaviors (objectives) identified, the next task is for the provider and/or staff to determine the frequency and type of interventions necessary to facilitate the behavioral change. Some terms often used instead of *interventions* are *methods, actions, approaches,* and *modalities.* When constructing this section of the plan of care, the following questions should be posed:

- What interventions (group, client, family, medication, and/or client assignments) are apt to be the most effective in maximizing the behavioral improvement of the client?
- How often should the intervention(s) be implemented? How great an intensity can the client tolerate?
- What discipline(s) or staff have the competence to implement them for this client? Who will be the staff responsible?

Through the screening or assessment process and continuing observations, staff remain aware of the qualitative responses of the client to care, treatment, or service. For 24-hour settings, they determine whether the client is apt to participate or remain isolated in group settings and whether sufficient cognitive abilities exist for the client to benefit from educational groups, computerized tutorials, or reading assignments. They determine what types of recreation or occupational therapy would be the most effective. In brief, they develop a process uniquely designed to address the specific needs and desires of the client. For community-based settings, data recording the clients' functioning in the community are continually assessed.

Interventions are an important part of the plan. The frequency of specific modalities (for example, job coaching, group, family, client sessions) should be delineated. The name of the client(s) or the discipline (for example, foster care coordinator, case manager, counselor) who will deliver them is required as well. The benefits of specificity will show themselves later during the progress review sessions, particularly when a client is not progressing as quickly as planned. During the session, it can be determined whether the client received the recommended number and type of interventions that were planned. If the services were not delivered as planned, the explanation for lack of progress might be evident. On the other hand, if the client received the recommended interventions and participated fully, there are ample data to determine if the type, frequency, or intensity should be increased or if new or different approaches might be necessary. Examples of interventions are shown in Sidebar 3-4 (page 59).

Sidebar 3-4

Interventions

- Client sessions, daily by psychologist
- Group therapy, daily by social worker
- Recreational activities, daily by trained staff
- Client will complete a first-step inventory.
- Medication (name) is administered by trained staff.
- Job coaching
- Parent skills training

After the plan has been completed and the interventions implemented, the next checkpoint is the timely review of the plan. When the plan has been skillfully developed, the review can generally be conducted according to the preestablished schedule. But if the condition of the client changes significantly—particularly if it worsens—the plan should be reviewed, regardless of the established schedule.

Whether it is scheduled or convened because of special need, the review session should be devoted to the evaluation of the progress of the client toward the achievement of the established objectives. If the client is making the changes as scheduled, nothing more may need to be done at that point. If the active problems/needs have been resolved, then different problems/needs from the list may be activated.

If the client is not progressing, a determination should be made as to whether the planned interventions were implemented. Did the client participate in the sessions? Did the recommended provider (or discipline) provide the care, or did other staff provide it? Were the medications administered as ordered? Did new issues arise that were not previously identified, thereby resulting in the need for a plan of care revision? Were there other problems that should have been pursued first or concurrently with the ones being reviewed?

If everything has been done in compliance with the plan, but the client is still not progressing as quickly as anticipated, a reassessment should be initiated to determine if the needs of the client have changed. If the needs have changed, then the new or additional care issues should be documented, using the same process that was used at the time of the initial assessments. If a problems/needs list is being used, the newly identified needs are to be inserted and prioritized. If there is a different mechanism for tracking the problems/needs of the client, it should be accessed and the new information added.

Making modifications to plans, backtracking, changing problems/needs statements, amending goals and objectives, revising the frequency and type of interventions, and assigning different providers are all positive and productive decisions. They reflect the dynamic nature of effective planning of care. Being human, clients do not always improve on a linear path; instead, they can move forward, fall backward, or deviate sideways. And the planning of care process is a continuous cycle, evolving as necessary based on the problems/needs of the client.

Providers should be realistic when establishing care goals and objectives. When reimbursement was less restricted, and care, treatment, and services less rigidly regulated, clients were freer to pursue long-term care goals for problems/needs that were not necessarily disabling but that did diminish the quality of their lives. Today, for many organizations, care is much more crisis focused and much briefer. Objectives focus on restoring the client to a functional state. At the very time that issues are more complicated, providers are expected to bring them under control more quickly than ever before, to salvage enough resources to treat additional complicated clients. Joint Commission surveyors have noted that many organizations have not modified their plans of care in accordance with the shorter lengths of stay. When unrealistic plans of care are written, clients do not meet many of their goals and objectives, and staff can therefore feel unsuccessful, which can lead to burnout and frustration.

Despite some very real constraints, all problems or needs of the client should be identified during assessment. Some may be deferred until later in the care cycle, and some referred to another provider. Some may simply disappear as other problems are resolved. With shorter lengths of stay, developing plans of care that take the continuity of care into account is critical. For instance, crisis stabilization units might limit their focus on crisis management, symptom stabilization, and after-care planning. The client may then be referred to other programs/services that focus on the following:

- Restoring or maintaining the functional abilities related to living, learning, and work activities
- Transitioning to more independent and less restrictive environments
- Successfully adapting into natural or community settings

Some organizations' scope of services may include only screening with referral(s) for full assessment(s).

THE STRUCTURE OF PLANNING OF CARE

To better understand how a plan of care is put together, refer to the written analysis for Mary in Section 2, page 37. A problems/needs list based on the written analysis summary was developed by collating the strengths and needs of the client from the physical, psychosocial, and spiritual assessments. The interdisciplinary plan of care for Mary is shown in Figure 3-5, page 61.

Participation of Clients

The client should actively participate in the planning of care process. Participation requires more than just having the client sign the plan (in fact, Joint Commission standards do not require that the client sign his or her plan of care). A signature denotes only that the client agreed to sign the plan; it does not reflect the contributions he or she made to its development or his or her responses to the goals and objectives. There should be some documentation in the record of the personal care goals and objectives of the client. Presumably, they will be congruent with the staff's goals.

The plan of care is not prepared based entirely on problems or deficits. The plan of care also considers the strengths of the client. In the case that follows, Mary is cognizant of her issues and needs and can participate in planning of care (that is, a habilitative approach). She can help establish priorities for care. She has a stable environment, work skills, and potential. There are no limiting financial issues. Finally, there do not appear to be any barriers to growth potential.

One method of reflecting the participation of the client is to include a specific progress note that summarizes the following:

- The degree to which the client was involved in planning of care

---

Figure 3-5

Ensuring that Documentation Remains Viable: Making Adjustments

Problem Number	Meeting Date: 1/20/XX

1A

Updated or New Problem: Physical Problem A—individual served is 40 pounds overweight.
Goal: To bring weight within average range according to height and age.
Objective:
Individual served will lose 5 pounds.
Interventions (including responsibility):
• 1,500 calorie diet—monitored by staff
• Dietary counseling twice weekly—by dietician
• Individual therapy three times weekly—by social worker
• Full participation in daily unit schedule—by case manager (monitor)

Anticipated Date of Achievement: 10/22/XX
Signature of Staff/Date: _____

1B

Updated or New Problem: Blood pressure 160/110.
Goal: To attain blood pressure within average range.
Objective:
To maintain blood pressure below 130/90.
Interventions (including responsibility):
• Relaxation therapy three times weekly—by activities therapist
• Individual counseling three times weekly—by social worker
• Medication per doctor's orders—by trained staff

Anticipated Date of Achievement: 10/15/XX
Signature of Staff/Date: _____

3A,B,E

Updated or New Problem: Depressed mood as evidenced by:
A. Sleeping only four hours per night
B. Overeating
E. Unable to identify positive things in her life
Goal: To be free of depression.
Objective(s):
A. Individual served will sleep at least eight hours per night without interruptions.
B. Individual served will consume 1,800 calories daily.
E. Individual served will identify five positive things in her current life.

Interventions (including responsibility):
A. Physical recreation one hour daily—by recreation staff
A. Insomniacs group once weekly—by psychologist
E. Written assignment, individual served to find one positive thing for each negative thing she identifies—by individual served and case manager

Anticipated Date of Achievement: A-10/22/XX; E-10/18/XX

Signature of Staff/Date: _____

Signature of Individual Served/Date: _____

This figure shows a sample interdisciplinary plan of care for Mary.

Source: Joint Commission Resources: *A Practical Guide to Documentation in Behavioral Health Care,* 2nd ed. Oakbrook Terrace, IL: The Joint Commission, 2002.

- The degree to which the client understands the plan of care
- The degree to which the client agrees with (or is committed to) the plan of care

This approach is reflected in the following example.

Progress Notes Summarizing the Participation of the Client

EXAMPLE Mary met with the team to discuss the plan of care. The identified problems, goals, and objectives were read, and she was asked for her reaction. She understood them, considered them realistic, and said that she would work on them. She expressed some reservation related to having her spouse involved during the assessments. She stated that she did not want any formal meetings with him but wanted him to visit as often as possible. The team agreed that even a preliminary formal joint session would not be advisable for at least two weeks. Mary signed the plan to formalize her approval.

Next, Mary met with the primary therapist to further discuss the plan of care. The identified problems, goals, and objectives were again read. She agreed to work on the problem related to isolating herself, but refused to work on the objective related to her family problems. The therapist advised her that the staff believed it was a significant problem but would defer working on it until she thought she was ready. Mary signed the plan and added her comments regarding the item with which she disagreed.

During the planning of care session, the responsible staff prioritizes the order in which the problems will be addressed. The decisions emerge from the collective wisdom of the care team—if the level of care allows for a team—or from the judgment of the assigned provider in care levels where teams do not exist. The prioritized problems are brought over to the planning of care form (*see* Figure 3-5, page 61).

The inclusion of forms in this book does not suggest that they should be used or, even more important, that they are useful for everyone. Determining the purpose of a form is far more important than its shape, design, or format. Before creating a new or different document, consider the form's purpose. It is surprising how many organizations create new forms to resolve problems rather than modifying the processes that created the problems.

As noted in Figure 3-5, the team decides to address Mary's physical issues and some of those related to her depressed mood. Each goal is logically linked to the identified problem. Each goal expresses in general terms what would demonstrate optimal resolution of the problem being addressed. The objectives are far more explicit. They are logically linked to the goal and the problem statement. From Mary's perspective, they are realistic and attainable.

In Sidebar 3-5 on page 63, one organization shares its experience with modifying and improving its forms to improve its process of documentation.

Progress Notes

Each time a progress note is entered into the clinical/case record, the staff member entering it should review the documented care objectives to determine what the intended note has to do with the plan of care. If a progress note bears no relationship to the plan of care, there may be some difficulties with either the plan or the note. If significant events are occurring in care, treatment, or services that require a progress note but are not associated with the plan, then the plan may need to be revised.

Sidebar 3-5

Ensuring That Documentation Remains Viable: Making Adjustments

At New Directions, a residential youth addictions organization based in Cleveland, Ohio, staff are always looking at ways to improve their documentation and how it aids them in their daily work. "We don't look at our documentation as being isolated from anything else we do at New Directions," notes Sue Tager, L.S.W., L.I.C.D.C., Performance Improvement and Program Standards coordinator at New Directions. "Our goal is to make sure our documentation is as effective as possible and that it works well with how we want to serve our clients." The policy at New Directions is, therefore, to make changes in its documentation approach if staff determine that making a change will help them more effectively meet their goals to provide excellent care, treatment, and services.

One regular and required activity for the youth at New Directions is a monthly drug screening. In the past, staff would receive the drug screen result and then be required to document in a progress note that they had met with the youth and shared the result with him or her. The staff would also then sign a form indicating that they had reviewed and reported the result. "We realized it was an extra step in our documentation, and while the progress note did state that the staff member had shown results to the youth, it was not always clear to verify what information the youth was given or how it was presented," Tager explains. Eventually, Tager modified the drug screen form to include the signature of the youth as well. "This way both the youth and staff member sign their receipt of these findings at the same time, we know that the youth has actually seen the results and there has been a discussion of these results, and we have one less piece of documentation to deal with."

 Check the CD-ROM: See "Urine Drug Screening Policy & Procedure" in the Appendix on the CD-ROM, for New Directions' policy and procedure that outlines this process.

Tager notes that New Directions' philosophy about handling documentation reflects the organization's overall approach to providing care, treatment, and services. "Everything we do is with the client at the forefront," she notes. "After all, the better our documentation is, the more we can know and the more we can do for the client. And isn't that better for the client? Isn't it worth it to do this for the clients?"

A progress note that does not relate to the plan may be written because a significant issue has emerged that should be added to the problems/needs list. If that is the case, a decision should be made as to whether the problem is to be activated and the existing plan revised. A second possibility is that the activity being recorded/documented had nothing to do with the plan of care. A third possibility is that the note was written to comply with an organization's expectation that a specific number of scheduled notes are written per day, per week, or per shift. The mandated volume rule occurs most often in the intense levels of care, treatment, or services in which organization rules and regulations, program plans, and policies and procedures demand a note on every shift for every client. At best, this can become a creative challenge for the staff, particularly for those working the night and early morning shifts. Unless the client is being treated for a sleep disorder, it is difficult to write relevant progress notes about sleeping clients.

As a consequence, reviews of clinical/case records may uncover benign progress notes, such as "Client slept through the night," "Client was restless through the night," or "Client in bed all night."

There is probably no way to make required progress notes more relevant. Supervisors might wish to review their requirements to determine whether such documentation requirements can be eliminated or reduced. Except for these obvious exceptions, progress notes should consistently communicate progress of the client toward attaining care objectives.

Writing progress notes serves as a semiformal plan of care review. The note should reflect evaluation of the progress of the client toward the care objectives. If the notes over time suggest no significant change or a worsening of the condition of the client, staff should seriously consider convening a special planning of care review session.

A progress note is intended to contain more than just anecdotal material. The primary purpose is to review the progress of the client in relation to the plan of care. Thus, each progress note becomes a short-term plan of care review.

One problem that providers often make is to write process notes rather than progress notes. Process notes typically are limited to what the client has said or done during the time the provider interacted with him or her. the following are examples of process notes:

- "Mark participated in group."
- "Helen said: 'I told my child that I would talk with him as soon as I was off the phone.'"
- "Joe was angry today."

Progress notes typically include some process information, but they also reflect the implementation of the plan, the behavioral changes in the client over time, the degree to which the objectives are being met, and any immediate changes to the plan. Providers need to document specific events/responses in a developmental context.

For Mark, the provider should document the quality of participation and whether his participation improves over time.

For Helen, the provider should document whether her response was appropriate and whether it reflected her application of a new parenting skill to her home environment.

For Joe, the provider should document how Joe expressed his anger, whether his response was an improvement from previous responses, and whether the response reflected the application of new anger management skills.

Not every progress note has to reflect all the components listed above. However, over time, progress notes should reflect the implementation of the plan, the response of the client, the degree to which the objectives are being met, and any planned changes. The Joint Commission does not specify how often progress notes should be documented, their content, or their format. Providers are responsible for determining each of those guidelines, based on the organization's mission, scope of services, and population(s) served.

Plan of Care Reviews

The formal plan of care review should be devoted to examining the active plan; the progress of the client in relation to the goals, objectives, and time frames; and the addition, deletion, or revision of goals, objectives, and interventions. If warranted, new problems can be added to the active plan, as well as measures to track and implement the strategies. If the plan of care has been subject to continuous mini-reviews and in-progress notes described earlier, the formal plan of care review should be neither time-consuming nor full of surprises. The checkpoint serves primarily as a formalization of the less structured reviews that occur continuously during staff interactions, change-of-shift reports, group and client therapy, community meetings, and all other situations in which interaction with the client occurs.

Joint Commission standards do not mandate specific review time frames. However, the standards require that the plan be evaluated periodically. The time frames of review should include regular intervals (for instance, at planning of care meetings) and be responsive to specific events (such as identification of a new significant problem/need, occurrence of a crisis, or lack of progress). Again, the review time frames need to be defined by each organization.

Discharge and Aftercare Planning

The process of managed care has significantly affected the structure of behavioral health care delivery. One of the most striking outcomes has been the expansion of continuum of planning of care, facilitating transfer to lower levels of care, treatment, or service as the acuity of the client's condition changes. The continuum of care requires the provider to establish mechanisms that will track the resolution of client problems over time. When the client is ready to move to a different program or service or to another provider, a plan for the continuation is necessary.

As noted in Section 2, one of the benefits of problems/needs lists is that they provide a convenient way of listing the multiple problems/needs a client may bring to care, treatment, or service. They permit a provider to identify which problems/needs have been satisfactorily resolved and which have yet to be addressed. They are most valuable at the time of completion of care, treatment, or services with the client because they permit easy identification of the remaining unresolved issues that require attention.

A characteristic of behavioral health care problems is that they develop over prolonged periods of time. Generally, anything that takes a long time to develop takes a long time to change. Time itself can be a factor in the healing process. However, during an era of restricted lengths of care, the ability to take care of a problem within a single level of care or by a single provider is diminished.

The discharge/aftercare planning process is the final phase of the planning of care. Remaining problems/needs are identified. Unresolved problems/needs requiring additional attention are prioritized. Depending on the nature of those problems/needs, continuing care providers with the competence to address the specific issues of the client are identified. Regardless of the number of remaining unresolved issues, there is usually one continuing care provider principally responsible for overseeing the continuing care of the client. This provider serves as case manager and invariably is a qualified provider. Any remaining problems/needs that do not require immediate attention are deferred to the provider who has agreed to coordinate the continuing care. The care team or case manager identifies providers capable of addressing those remaining issues and contacts them about their willingness and ability to provide the recommended care. Their names, addresses, e-mail addresses, and phone numbers are recorded and included in the continuing plan of care. Whenever possible, a scheduled appointment is made and reflected as part of the continuing care process.

In many instances, problems/needs associated with the family, job, and other support systems may not require formal interventions. They improve as a natural outcome of the improvement of the client. There may also be problems/needs that had to be deferred during the most recent care episode and must be referred again now that completion of care, treatment, or services is imminent.

When the problems or needs have been prioritized and the continuing care providers identified, the client and assigned provider meet to review the proposed plan. Whenever possible, the family should participate in the discussion because family members will most likely serve as the main support system of the client. The family should understand and be educated about the continuing plan of care, particularly when medication is recommended. They should be reasonably informed about the type of medication, the importance of its continued use, its effects, any potential hazards, possible side effects, appropriate dosages, and frequency of administration.

The importance of the discharge or aftercare planning session for a behavioral health care problem cannot be overemphasized. Public sentiment is still not fully supportive of the concept of emotional problems/needs as health issues. Families are not necessarily apt to openly or comfortably acknowledge behavioral health care problems or needs afflicting family members to neighbors, friends, or even other family members. Attitudes, although improving, can still include guilt, shame, and embarrassment.

Clients may be strongly motivated to abandon care, treatment, or services as quickly as possible if only because the absence of care implies the absence of illness. The client and family may have to be persuaded that ongoing care, treatment, or service is valuable or even critical. Because resistance may be strong—although hidden and perhaps even unconscious—preparation generally starts early in the care process. Most providers state that continuing planning of care begins at the onset of care, but this statement is often more a slogan than a practice.

Discharge or aftercare planning should discuss how the client and/or family can access care again if it becomes necessary. As with any health condition, clients are hopeful—perhaps even convinced—that there will not be a need for further care, treatment, or services. Because many behavioral health problems or needs are chronic or recurring, it may be beneficial to teach the client and family how to reenter the system, preferably before things get so bad that a more intense level of care, treatment, or service is required.

There are several methods used to document a continuing plan of care. When a client is being transferred from one program or service to another, a transfer summary is usually the preferred format. The transfer summary concisely identifies the condition of the client upon onset of care, the problems/needs that were treated, the response of the client, and the condition of the client at the point of transfer. The record will follow the client, so the problems/needs list and/or analysis of the assessment data will be available to the staff at the new program or service.

When clients are leaving one provider to go to another, there are at least two methods of documenting the continuing plan of care. The first is to include it in the discharge summary/clinical résumé. The Joint Commission requires that every discharge summary include the content listed in Sidebar 3-6, below. Some providers, in order to track outcomes and maximize client improvement, develop a separate continuing plan of care, similar to the one in Sidebar 3-7, page 67. Some behav-

---

Sidebar 3-6

Discharge Summary/Clinical Résumé Contents

At discharge, a discharge summary/clinical résumé concisely summarizes the following:
- The reason for care or service
- The significant findings
- Procedures performed and care, treatment, or service rendered
- Condition of the client at discharge or transfer
- Specific instructions (aftercare or continuing plan of care) given to the client and/or family

---

Sidebar 3-7

Continuing Plan of Care

The first example appearing in Section 2 (*see* page 20) presents the case of a 30-year-old woman who was sexually abused as a youth, has a lifelong history of alcohol and substance abuse, and has had several very traumatic experiences. A primary concern is that she is suicidal. Her plan of care addresses these issues, and competent clinical staff work with her to resolve suicidal ideation and complete a rehabilitation program for alcohol and drug abuse. Initial issues of trauma are addressed. In preparing a discharge plan, staff recognize the self-esteem problems related to her sexual abuse and the impact of this on her long-term alcohol and drug abuse. They recognize that she would need a year or more of client counseling with a counselor who works with abused women. The referral for this case is the first part of the continuing plan of care. Staff also recognize that she will need to work through several issues with a trauma group over the next year. This is the second part of the continuing plan of care. Lifelong work with Alcoholics Anonymous or a similar program may be necessary as well, which would be the final part of her continuing plan of care.

---

ioral health care does not result in discharge, such as opioid addiction treatment programs and some services to persons with developmental disabilities.

In Sidebar 3-8 (page 68), Hillel Bodek, M.S.W., L.C.S.W.-R, B.C.D., a clinical social worker in private practice in New York and president of the New York State Society of Clinical Social Work, outlines the elements that should be included in an interval or closing/termination summary. Although this has been written for those who work in the field of clinical social work, the principles can provide important guides for all types of behavioral health care settings.

Practice Guidelines

A practice guideline describes the processes used to evaluate and treat a client having a specific diagnosis, condition, or symptom. Practice guidelines are found in the literature under many names: *clinical practice guidelines, practice parameters, care protocols, standards of practice, clinical pathways, care maps,* and other descriptive terms. In all cases, guidelines should be evidence based and shown to be efficacious and effective within defined populations or services. If a provider uses a practice guideline, he or she should be certain to individualize that guideline for the client in order to reflect individualized planning of care. As computerization of records becomes more sophisticated, practice guidelines will be tailored much more easily to the individualized needs of the clients. The use of such a practice guideline is acceptable if it is developed after the other assessments have been completed, thereby permitting a blending of information, and if it references each aspect—physical, psychosocial, and others—as appropriate.

DEFINING COMPETENCIES

Except in nursing, very little emphasis is placed on the value or necessity of documentation during professional preparation. Even less attention is paid to teaching the techniques. As a result, new graduates rely on peers or supervisors who have learned from their own mentors. As a result, poor documentation can become a generational legacy.

Sidebar 3-8

Elements of an Appropriate Interval or Closing/Termination Summary

An interval or closing/termination summary, which may be abbreviated or elongated depending on the circumstances of a particular case, documents the clinician's thoughtful reflection on the clinical course of the client's treatment (to date in relation to an interval summary, or with regard to the entire period of treatment in relation to a closing/termination summary). Such summaries can be useful if the client later seeks treatment from another clinician and requests that a summary be sent to that clinician. The documentation of a proper interval or closing/termination summary includes the following:

1. The dates the client was referred, first contacted the clinician, and was first seen; the referral source; and the time period covered by the summary (if this is a closing/termination summary, the date the client was last seen and the last contact with the client)

2. A synopsis of the initial reason for and background circumstance of the referral, the presenting problem(s) from the client's perspective at intake, the client's initial clinical presentation, and the initial assessment, including the initial diagnoses and initial identified problem(s) as identified by the practitioner

3. A review of the problem areas and symptoms addressed in treatment, the treatment modalities used, the client's clinical course in treatment during the treatment period in question (noting changes, if any, in the client's symptoms, thinking, emotions, beliefs, behaviors, and other areas of biopsychosocial functioning), and the extent that the identified symptoms/problems were resolved and the treatment goals established were achieved during the treatment period in question

4 A summary of any concurrent treatments (including the provider[s] of such treatments, the names and dosages of medications prescribed, other treatments rendered, or any other relevant assessments performed), the steps taken to coordinate care with other practitioners (including the extent and success of achieving collaboration, or any problems that interfered with collaborative efforts), and the impact/results of the other concurrent treatments

5. If this is a closing/termination summary, a statement regarding the circumstances of the termination of treatment (precipitants—Was it planned or unplanned? Was it mutually agreed upon by client and the clinician? Did the client stop coming and, if so, what steps were taken to address this and with what results?)

6. If this is a closing/termination summary, include final diagnoses and a statement as to the client's functioning, as well a statement as to which, if any, of the concurrent treatments (including medication) the client is receiving, those the client intends to continue (if so, from whom and to what extent), and those the client does not intend to continue (if so, include the client's reasons for discontinuation of those services)

7. If there is a closing/termination summary, a statement detailing any referrals or recommendations provided to the client regarding further care, and the client's response to such referrals and recommendations

8. If there is a closing/termination summary, a statement of whether the client poses a risk of decompensation, suicidality, assaultiveness, homicidality, relapse back to alcoholism or substance abuse, inability to care for himself or herself, of being victimized, of victimizing others, or is at any other serious risk at the time of termination/closing; the basis of the risk assessment; details of the steps taken to address any of these risks; and the results of such steps

Source: Excerpted and summarized from "Standards for Clinical Documentation and Recordkeeping," by Hillel Bodek, M.S.W., L.C.S.W.-R, B.C.D. © 2003, 2006, 2007. Used with permission. Permission to reproduce for educational purposes is granted provided attribution is included.

One of the greatest hurdles interfering with documentation competence is overcoming the staff's belief that there has to be a difference between how one thinks, acts, and talks, and how care, treatment, or services are documented.

Questions asked about staff competencies are similar to those asked about the outcomes of clients. The question asked about clients is "What does a client have to do (that is, behaviorally) to demonstrate that he or she is achieving objectives?" The critical question asked about staff and their competence is "What does a staff member have to do to demonstrate that he or she is achieving performance objectives?"

Competence can be partially determined through review of clinical/case records. The greater the congruence between how providers perform and how well they document that performance, the more accurately reviews of clinical/case records will validate their competence. Also, review Section 2, pages 17–48, for additional tips on improving documentation skills and competency.

A universal performance standard for professionals should be the ability to use the clinical/case record of the client as a technique. Each provider will have to establish special standards. They will vary because of the uniqueness of the mission, values, and philosophy of each organization and of its staffing patterns. Examples of how documentation expectations can be used as performance standards are shown in Sidebar 3-9, page 70. The reader is cautioned that these are examples and are not intended to be prescriptive or considered to be applicable to all providers. The underlying concepts are of greatest importance. Competence can be best evaluated through the direct observation of behaviors.

MANAGING THE PROCESS OF CHANGE IN DOCUMENTATION

Sometimes changes in documentation processes are driven by the organization (such as when a decision is made to change or offer new services), and sometimes they are driven by external factors (such as new requirements from regulating bodies or reimbursement sources). Often organization-driven change allows for more flexibility in when and how modifications are made and how they are implemented, but when changes need to be made for the purpose of complying with new regulations or requirements, organizations have to act nimbly and effectively to ensure that the changes happen in a timely manner, often because of specific effective dates imposed by these outside agencies. For example, the Lake County Health Department and Community Health Center's Behavioral Health Services, based in Waukegan, Illinois, faced a series of coding changes from the state that mandated an effective and rapid response to ensure that its documentation met the new requirements. In Sidebar 3-10, pages 71–72, Lake County Health Department shares its experiences with adjusting its organization, its staff, and its documentation to a new set of expectations from the State of Illinois.

JOINT COMMISSION REQUIREMENTS AND STANDARDS RELATING TO DOCUMENTATION

The implicit expectation for documentation permeates the entire body of Joint Commission standards and requirements. The majority of specific requirements, particularly as they relate to documentation for screening, assessment, planning of care, reassessment, discharge planning, and so on, appears primarily in two of the standards chapters: the "Provision of Care, Treatment, and Services" chapter and the "Management of Information" chapter. Additional documentation-related standards and requirements appear in the National Patient Safety Goals, the "Leadership" chapter, and the "Improving Organization Performance" chapters. Although these standards chapters do undergo revisions and updates, the requirements remain consistent with the principle of ensuring

---

Sidebar 3-9

Components of Good Documentation

- **Physical Examination**
  The physical examination documents the following:
  - Review of systems
  - Family medical history
  - Medical history of the client
  - Substance abuse history of the client and his or her family
  - Evaluation of results in language that is understandable to the client and nonmedical staff
  - Recommendations for medical care, treatment, or services
  - Interpretation of the overall physical condition of the client and its implications for his or her specific behavioral health care issues

- **Analysis of Assessment Data**
  The assigned provider documents the following:
  - Evaluation of physical, psychological, and social status of the client
  - Strengths and needs (that is, problems) of the client
  - Evaluation in observable behavioral terms

- **Continuing Plan of Care/Discharge Plan/Clinical Résumé**
  The assigned provider documents the following:
  - Remaining problems to be referred
  - Participation in planning by the client and his or her family, as appropriate
  - Name, address, e-mail address, and phone number of the primary continuing care provider and all other scheduled caregivers, and the date and time of the first appointment with that provider(s)

- **Plan of Care**
  Contributors document the following:
  - Problem statements in terms of observable behaviors of the client
  - Strengths and problems/needs of the client
  - Objectives in terms of desired, improved, observable, and measurable client behaviors
  - Target dates for achievement of each objective
  - Individualized discharge criteria, if discharge is appropriate
  - Interventions by modality, frequency, and assigned provider

---

precise, well-planned, and accurate documentation for clients served in order to ensure the delivery of safe, high-quality care, treatment, and services.

Organizations should review the requirements outlined in the *Comprehensive Accreditation Manual for Behavioral Health Care* (*CAMBHC*), any federal requirements, and any additional specific requirements or regulations outlined for them by the states in which they provide services to ensure that their documentation meets these guidelines. As mentioned in Section 1 (pages 1–16), regulatory agencies in some states (for example, Ohio) have begun offering a streamlined, standardized series of

Sidebar 3-10

Managing Change in Documentation at a Community Mental Health Center

Lake County Health Department and Community Health Center's Behavioral Health Service (LCHD/BHS) has been providing behavioral health care services to the local population in multiple locations in Lake County, Illinois, for many years and is familiar with the need for and benefit of effective documentation in providing that care. When the State of Illinois announced its release of revisions to Medicaid Rule 132, changes in documentation for assessment and reassessment were required. Therefore, the LCHD, and any other Illinois agencies receiving reimbursement for providing behavioral health care under Medicaid, needed to make changes to a number of their forms. Some of the organization's most frequently used forms would have to be changed, and the process required a planned and organized approach, including a communication strategy and education. It also required that key staff members take on leadership roles to help coordinate and guide the changes so that they could be in place by the state's effective date of October 1, 2007. Also, because some of the changes had to be in place by July 1, 2007, the process had to follow a two-stage schedule.

After attending training and informational sessions provided by the State of Illinois, managers from the LCHD/BHS reconvened in their organization to determine the best approach to educating staff, making necessary changes, and implementing the changes by the deadlines. The group determined that one staff member should be the key point person to help guide and coordinate the process toward completion. This role was taken on by Kathie Kostock, L.C.S.W., Outpatient Mental Health Adult Services coordinator at the LCHD/BHS. Kostock found that specific steps in the process required a group of decisions and other steps benefited from having fewer individuals actively involved in making the specific changes but having a review note.

"We went through the summary of changes outline, as well as the new rule that we downloaded from the Internet," Kostock explains. "Our database manager had to go through the guidelines and updated our codes and reimbursement amounts and new codes were added. We compared our Daily Activity Schedule codes manual as well as forms and indentified changes. We also had to work with those programs that had new codes that were required to be in documentation and on the treatment plans by July 1." The LCHD also had to ensure that specifically required applications were made to the state on a timely basis.

Because changes to actual forms often also require updating related policies and procedures, Kostock then updated all of the related policies and sent drafts to multiple reviewers for feedback. Several staff then piloted the use of some of the forms to determine what, if any, modifications needed to be made for formatting or content, which is essential when making large-scale changes. Kostock explains, "We decided it would be hard for staff to track the date of an annual update of the assessment, and we felt compliance would be more consistent and meet a higher quality standard if we did it twice a year."

Navigating this update process required regular communication with all staff so that they were prepared for the new changes and would be able to use the revised forms as easily as possible. Kostock sent regular e-mails to staff to keep them apprised of changes. In these e-mails Kostock highlighted the key issues that staff needed to know and provided them with additional information and resources in case

(continued)

Sidebar 3-10 (continued)

they needed more guidance. She also provided educational materials to managers so that they could in turn train and work with their own staff on understanding and using the new forms. *See* Figure 3-6, below, for an example of an e-mail Kostock sent to staff to give them updates and provide education on upcoming changes, and *see* Figure 3-7, pages 73–74, for an educational memorandum shared with staff to ensure that they had the right information about changes in documentation.

Figure 3-6

Example of an E-mail Communicating Documentation Changes

From:	Kostock, Kathleen M.
To:	HL BHS Users
Subject:	NEW ASSESSMENT FORMS ARE READY!!! Read the Attachments!
Importance:	High
Attachments:	Assessment Education Memo.doc; HOW TO USE DROP.doc

Dear Staff,

The new assessment forms are ready and available on the U drive. **The implementation date is Monday, October 1, 2007.** Please stop using old hand-written and computer forms. Make copies of the templates listed in the memo below to your Y drive or make copies of the hand-written forms.

Instruction Memo: **Instructions on How to Use Drop-Downs:**

Assessment   HOW TO USE
|ucation Memo.do   DROP.doc (31 KE

If you have any questions, please let me know.

Kathie

Kathleen M. Kostock, LCSW
Outpatient Mental Health Services Coordinator
Lake County Health Department and Community Health Center
Behavioral Health Services

A sample memo used to communicate documentation changes.

Source: Lake County Health Department and Community Health Center, Behavioral Health Services, Waukegan, IL. Used with permission.

Sidebar 3-10 (continued)

Figure 3-7

Example of Educational Memorandum Outlining Changes in Documentation

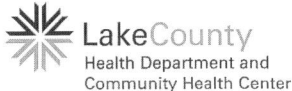 LakeCounty
Health Department and
Community Health Center

Behavioral Health Services

MEMORANDUM

DATE: September 25, 2007

TO: BHS Staff

FROM: Kathie Kostock

RE: Revised and New Assessment Templates

During the past several months MH and CD Steering Committees have met and reviewed the new Medicaid Rule 132 and DASA standards in the area of assessment and re-assessment and revised our current assessment forms. *Please remove old hand-written forms from shelves, and drawers as well as computer forms from your Y drive. These forms are effective 10-01-07.* There are hand and computer/drop-down forms available on U/BH/All BHS Staff/Forms/Forms C&H. The following forms have been revised to meet the new standards:

- Comprehensive Assessment-Adult
- Comprehensive Assessment-Child and Adolescent
- Initial Assessment-Adult

The following are the main changes to the three forms:

1. In the Document Section-the title of the form was shortened to Comprehensive Assessment-Adult for the Adult form.
2. The Financial Resources was moved to the Identifying Information Section of the Initial Assessment to mirror the Comprehensive Assessment.
3. Medical History was consolidated into one section with the name of the client's primary Care Physician and their contact information added. Also added was a check box to note that consent form was in the chart.
4. In the section that notes the reviewing the Health Screening the section for pain, nutrition and dental were added.
5. History of Mental Health Treatment was consolidated. Outcome was added as a prompt to length of treatment for inpatient and outpatient history. The date of the most recent psychiatric evaluation was added. The section regarding medication was broken out for previous, current as well as whether the client adheres to a medication regimen.
6. Chemical Dependency History title was changed to Alcohol & or Other Drug Use/Addiction History. A check box section was added for SAP Programs that use the SAP addendum instead of the text and drop-downs in this section. Also what was added was a section on the client's history of withdrawal symptoms, number of relapses, and history of prior alcohol & or Other drug screenings or evaluations.
7. In the family of origin/current family dynamics, the age when significant loses occurred.
8. In the Section Client's Personal Safety what was added was factors placing the client's family at risk.
9. A longer prompt was added to the Cultural/Ethnic Supports Issues section.

(continued)

Sidebar 3-10 (continued)

Figure 3-7 (continued)

10. A more detailed prompt was added to the Spiritual Supports/Issues
11. Under the Vocation Section that lists learning needs, the prompt Job readiness/barriers to employment was added. List daily activities if not employed was also added.
12. A more detailed Mental Status was added to the Initial Assessment.
13. The Clinical Summary and Diagnostic Impressions Section were changed to have the prompts that had been under the title of the section listed vertically. There are sections for: Integration of the information in the assessment including mental status as well as CD programs address all 6 ASAM criteria; 2) Stating the rationale for the DSM-IV diagnoses and clinical problems being addressed; 3) Client Desired Outcome of Treatment (Hopes, Dreams and Goals); 4) Strengths and Resources, willingness to participate in treatment; 5) Analysis of client's limitations and barriers to treatment inclusive needed case management to reduce identified barriers (i.e. childcare, transportation, living conditions health needs, etc.)
14. Under staff signature, Supervisor was added next to the QMHP signature for CD programs and language was added to the policy about after reviewing the assessment for medical/clinical necessity that the LPHA/MD signs and if applicable, records the date of the face-to-face-contact with the client.

The following are *new forms for Mental Health Programs Only:*

- Clinical Review-Adult
- Clinical Review-Child and Adolescent

1. The Clinical Review-Adult is a new form that reviews the client's response to treatment goals and objectives on the treatment plan, and updates the client's history and status in the areas of severity of illness, symptoms, changes in biomedical condition, current functional level, treatment acceptance or resistance, intensity of their service needs, steps towards mental health recovery, relapse potential for substance abuse and their current family/psychosocial environment and any changes in diagnosis. This update is completed at minimum every six months at the time the treatment plan is updated.
2. A Progress Note should document the DAS code of 114 for QMHP staff and 112 for MHP staff with the date, time, and location. The title of the progress note should be Clinical Review. It is filed in the continuum section of the chart.

PLEASE NOTE:

- *MH Programs will no longer use the Treatment Plan Progress Assessment Form. CD Programs that are currently using the Treatment Plan Progress Assessment will continue to do so.*
- *Programs who use the Initial Assessment form will continue to use the Psychosocial Assessment form prior to the development of the Treatment Plan.*
- *When doing an addendum on an existing treatment plan, a progress note should be completed documenting the need for additional goals, objectives and interventions. The Clinical Review form is only completed on the six month review date when the entire plan is updated.*

Thanks for your support in making these changes. If staff needs assistance in learning how to use the drop-down areas in the computer versions, (lock and unlock function) please let me know. Drop downs can be customized for your program for staff name or other program specific needs.

An example of a memo outlining changes in documentation used by the Lake County Health Department and Community Health Center.

Source: Lake County Health Department and Community Health Center, Behavioral Health Services, Waukegan, IL. Used with permission.

Sidebar 3-10 (continued)

No change on this scale unfolds in a perfectly smooth or predictable manner, and Kostock points to some interesting lessons learned along the way. "It can be challenging when you are making many changes, as it usually has to fall on only a few to do the majority of the work due to how detailed and tedious it can be," Kostock explains. But she notes that the concerted efforts undertaken by herself and her colleagues to ensure that changes were made in a thorough, detailed, and consistent manner helped the process move along as well as possible. She also offers the following lessons learned to any other organizations that may be required to make major changes in documentation due to changes in external regulations or requirements:

✓ Be patient. Undertaking and implementing major changes will take time and persistence, and above all it will require patience: Not everyone accepts and adjusts to change in the same way. Make sure that you take all the time you need to help staff adjust to the changes, and make sure that they feel empowered to ask questions along the way.

✓ Ask for input from key stakeholders. Any plans to make changes to documentation—particularly those used by staff on a regular basis—need to accommodate input from the staff who use them most frequently. Consider creative ways of asking for their input through such activities as surveys, direct interviews, or staff meetings.

✓ Don't expect everyone to give you feedback. In a perfect world, every staff member and key stakeholder will provide timely and helpful feedback, but that is not always a realistic goal in a busy organization that is on a deadline to implement changes. Keeping in mind that many changes such as these are driven by externally imposed deadlines, try to plan well enough in advance that you can secure feedback from as many staff as possible, but factor in a well-advertised cutoff date for feedback so you are not held back or unacceptably delayed.

✓ Critiques are not personal. Part of fostering a feedback process is embracing the concept that critiques are not directed at the persons involved in revising the process but are directed toward the changes being made. It can be challenging for the authors of changes in a process—be it documentation or anything else—to not form some degree of personal attachment to the work that is being done, but it is important and helpful to remember that the feedback being offered is and should be directed to the specific changes.

✓ Everyone has a certain level of stress during major changes. Individuals react differently to change, and when change is major and impacts many areas of an organization, it can cause a lot of stress for some staff members. Keep this in mind while planning for change and consider creative ways to help mitigate the stress by adding fun elements to the change process (such as including games in education sessions, holding parties to coincide with a launch or to acknowledge key milestones in the process, and so on).

✓ Pilot revised or new forms with a few key staff members to get accurate feedback. Take advantage of knowledgeable staff to help test the revised forms and give you feedback. Tap into a broad spectrum of staff, from the staff who have been with the organization and used the previous forms for a long time to the staff who may be new to the organization and who bring a different perspective to what may work well due to their experiences elsewhere. Piloting should also take place with different kinds of staff from different disciplines.

✓ Read your new rules or laws—do not interpret; if you are uncertain about something, get direct feedback from the state department that you are working with. If the changes to

(continued)

Sidebar 3-10 (continued)

documentation are being driven by a state or other regulating agency, always go to that source for guidance and additional interpretation on anything that is unclear. Most agencies and accrediting organizations will provide ways to get clarification on any unclear areas. Obtaining such clarification can prevent the stress and extra effort required to revise work already completed but based on incorrect assumptions about a rule or regulation.

With all of these newly revised changes only recently implemented at the LCHD, Kostock and her colleagues are still in the early days of seeing the impact of adapting to new forms throughout the organization and seeing what, if any, further changes may need to be made. "As we have only just launched the use of these new forms, we are still seeing if we need to offer additional training sessions and mentoring," she notes. They are also collecting feedback and observing any noticeable issues with using the forms so they can integrate that into any necessary updates. With the decision made early on to schedule regular updates to the forms and to involve as many staff at the right points along the way, Kostock feels that they will be able to make any necessary changes quickly and effectively as they become more accustomed to the new process in the coming months. "We are still learning about this process and expect to learn even more in time," Kostock notes. But with a successful and timely launch of these changes, combined with a dedicated and thorough approach to revising the forms, staff at the LCHD are well on their way to settling in to using the new forms without impairing their ability to provide high-quality, safe care to their clients.

 Check the CD-ROM: For examples of the revised assessment forms developed by the LCHD referred to in this sidebar, please see the Appendix on the companion CD-ROM.

---

forms that include all requirements and regulations that would apply to organizations in those states. These forms allow the organizations to save valuable time and resources that might otherwise have been used in trying to sort through the various regulations individually.

Currently under way is a concerted effort by The Joint Commission to improve the language, applicability, and relevance of its standards. The Joint Commission's Standards Improvement Initiative has been launched to accomplish the following for the behavioral health care standards beginning in 2008, with changes taking effect beginning in 2009:

- Clarify standards language.
- Ensure that standards are program specific.
- Delete redundant or nonessential standards.
- Consolidate similar standards.

In addition, the Joint Commission plans to reorganize the standards manuals, and the scoring and decision process will be refined. Beginning in 2008, the Joint Commission will seek feedback on standards for the behavioral health care accreditation programs.[1]

Documentation During the On-Site Survey

During the on-site accreditation survey, documentation is often taken into consideration by the Joint Commission. In Sidebar 3-11 (pages 77–79), Joint Commission surveyor Ben Lewis outlines some of his observations about documentation and what organizations should consider when working to improve their own processes.

Sidebar 3-11

The Surveyor Perspective on Documentation

During an on-site survey, surveyors need to navigate documentation while they trace clients and systems. Documentation plays a critically important role in outlining the experiences of that client while under the care, treatment, and services of the organization. It helps the surveyor identify what issues the clients face, what plan of care the organization has in place for those clients, and how the plan of care is being implemented. It links them to issues that may come up during tracer activities. Beyond problems with standards compliance and reimbursement, ineffective documentation can hinder effective planning of care and assessment, which can compromise the provision of safe, high-quality care, treatment, and services. In addition, the high rate of staff turnover in some areas of behavioral health care or the movement of clients among care settings means that in some ways documentation may be the vehicle that captures a solid history and background for a client. This is why the surveyor will often pay close attention to an organization's documentation.

Although surveyors do not conduct surveys with any expectation that all organizations have the same exact or standardized approach to documentation, there are some key consistent elements that they take into consideration while looking at documentation against the backdrop of the standards themselves. Does the documentation meet the expectations outlined in the standards? Does the process of documentation take into consideration an appropriate and timely assessment process? Does the documentation outline effective planning of care? Are the multidisciplinary elements of the assessment and planning of care process well integrated? Does the documentation really paint an accurate picture of the client and his or her needs and progress? What elements of discharge are integrated into the documentation and how is it mapped?

Documentation is not the key focus of a surveyor's assessment, but it does play an important role in their tracer activity. Ben Lewis, Ed.D., a surveyor with The Joint Commission for the behavioral health care program, notes that while many behavioral health care professionals possess sophisticated verbal skills and bring technical knowledge and expertise to their team discussions when planning care for a client, sometimes what is discussed quite astutely in team meetings is not always communicated properly in the documentation that he reviews. "Our clinicians often have excellent verbal skills," he explains. "But the documentation does not always match this." He notes that often while reviewing a record, he will have to ask additional questions to clarify an issue or understand what is meant. "The clinicians will have covered these issues in depth during treatment planning sessions, but will not translate that as well into the written form." He suggests that additional training and competency-building in documentation skills could help an organization create better, more comprehensive records for clients, which should improve the overall delivery of care, treatment, and services. Lewis attributes some of this lack of skill in written documentation to the fact that clinicians are not always provided with appropriate training during their academic education. He also notes that while some clinical professions do provide some training in documentation, others do not; this disparate approach can cause an inconsistency in the quality of documentation.

Coupled with the lack of written documentation training is the emergence of new technologies and increased redundancies in documentation, which Lewis feels are having an impact on the overall quality of documentation.

Lewis notes that while the introduction of electronically-based documentation systems can help streamline and speed up documentation for busy clinicians and have a positive impact on the delivery

(continued)

Sidebar 3-11 (continued)

of care, he warns against eliminating all written documentation. "Sometimes with the advent of electronic documentation, it is tempting to create forms that ask for data but don't ask for a lot of written documentation—this results in them being little more than a list of checkboxes," he explains. But Lewis's concern is that electronic documentation may omit the actual narrative about the client and his or her needs and evolving plan of care, making it more challenging to glean a solid understanding of that client. "We are pretty good at collecting a lot of data points about a client, but we are not focusing as much on pulling together a comprehensive textually driven picture of that client as well." So Lewis advises that in the process of implementing electronic systems, it is important to ensure that those systems still support the collection of the right data and documentation that ensures the best possible provision of care, treatment, and services.

At the other end of the spectrum is another area of concern for Lewis: redundancy in documentation. He notes that in the push to provide documentation from all possible disciplines in a particular organization (nursing, social work, and so on), the same data is sometimes collected on several forms. A multidisciplinary approach to care is far better for the client, Lewis stresses, but sometimes the actual approach to documentation in a multidisciplinary context ends up causing unwanted redundancies. He has often noticed when reviewing a client's record that some sections of a particular discipline's assessment may remain incomplete, or the same assessment is noted on four different forms. Lewis says that these organizations are asking for an assessment from their various disciplines but are often asking them to assess the same issues. "In some cases, staff will leave a section blank with the expectation that another discipline will fill in their part," Lewis explains. This omitted material can prove challenging to organizations if they are hoping to have complete and comprehensive information. Lewis advises that as organizations move more and more toward a multidisciplinary team approach, they should ensure that the documentation supports that approach as well. He suggests that organizations take some time to carefully review all of the documentation provided to ensure that there are no unnecessary redundancies, allowing staff to include more discipline-specific documentation and enabling them to focus on documenting those elements that are truly crucial to providing care.

Lewis offers the following suggestions to help organizations improve their documentation skills:

✓ Train the staff on improving documentation, but make it fun. When training and mentoring staff to improve their documentation skills, make it a productive and beneficial experience, but make it fun. "In trainings I've done, we would make it fun by using examples like Santa Claus as the client," notes Lewis. "We would give him a bipolar disorder." When trainings have an element of fun to them, it can be easier for staff to absorb the material while applying their knowledge to something whimsical. It can also aid with retention of knowledge.

✓ Make sure that the documentation accommodates what is being asked for. Lewis notes, "I have occasionally reviewed forms where a very profound question about the client is being asked—a question that may require a fairly substantial response—and the form only allows one or two lines for an answer." Providing forms that allow for appropriate responses can help ensure that the documentation meets the organization's goals.

✓ Don't forget the narrative. Lewis recommends that no matter what, the client's record should always include a narrative on the client. Much like what is discussed in planning and progress sessions, the client's documentation should also include a textual discussion of progress, needs, strengths, and planning. In case of staff turnover, this can be particularly

---

Sidebar 3-11 (continued)

important because the documentation may be the only source of information about a client if a staff member has left the organization.

Documentation can seem to be an additional, burdensome activity for staff to undertake while busy treating and caring for clients, but Lewis stresses that it can and should be regarded as the central repository of information, progress, and guidance for each client and as such is an important element of the care treatment process. How an organization manages its documentation can help determine its success in delivering safe, high-quality care, treatment, and services.

SUMMARY

The process of planning for care, treatment, and services is a natural outcome of the assessment process. It is a fluid system that requires continuous monitoring. If the monitoring is carried out effectively and efficiently, there should be no dramatic surprises during the course of care, treatment, or service, and even if there are, systems will be in place to make effective, midcourse adjustments. If conducted well, planning of care will truly drive the process. As clients change, plans will change. As plans change, clients will change.

An important function of the system is preparing the client and his or her family for continuing care to maximize the gains made during care, treatment, or service. Education about the nature of behavioral health problems/needs, particularly their tendency to recur unless the client and family heed the recommendations of professionals, is critical to the rehabilitation process.

Documentation performance standards are observable. They can be used by supervisors or by peers. Inferences can be made about the quality of care, treatment, or service in some instances based on the content of the clinical/case record. Organizations should consider convening documentation teams to establish performance standards and expectations.

REFERENCE

1. The Joint Commission: *Standards Improvement Initiative.* 2007. http://www.jointcommission.org/Standards/SII/ (accessed Oct. 26, 2007).

Glossary of Terms

Addiction Services/Programs

Behavioral health care services/programs for the assessment and/or care, treatment, or service of individuals with addictive behaviors, such as substance abuse, chemical dependency, or gambling.

Administration

The fiscal and general management of an organization, as distinct from the direct provision of care, treatment, or service.

Advocate

A person who represents the rights and interests of another client as though they were the person's own in order to realize the rights to which the client is entitled; obtain needed care, treatment, or service; and remove barriers to meeting the needs of the client.

Analysis of Assessment Data

An analysis of data gathered from the physical, psychological, social, and spiritual (as appropriate) assessments used to facilitate identification and prioritization of individual needs and to help determine the care and services to be provided.

Appropriateness

The degree to which the care provided is relevant to the individual's clinical needs, given the current state of knowledge.

Art Therapy

The use of art and artistic processes specifically selected and administered by an art therapist to restore, maintain, or improve an individual's mental, emotional, or social functioning.

Assess

To transform data into information by analyzing the data.

Assessment

The systematic collection and review of individual-specific data. The process established by an organization for obtaining appropriate and necessary information about each individual seeking entry into a health care setting or service. The information is used to match the needs of the client with the appropriate setting and intervention. An evaluation of history, tests, consultations, and any other data collected for the purpose of determining client strengths and needs. An assessment is not an abbreviated version of the client history.

Authenticate

To verify that an entry is complete, accurate, and final.

Availability

The degree to which appropriate care, treatment, and services are available to meet the needs of the client.

Behavior

The thoughts, feelings, beliefs, and/or actions of the client.

Behavioral Health Care

The continuum of psychosocial rehabilitation services that address a wide range of the needs of clients. This includes a broad array of mental health, foster care, forensic, chemical dependency, services for persons with developmental disabilities, and cognitive rehabilitation services provided in such care settings as acute, long term, and ambulatory.

Behavior Management

The use of basic learning techniques, such as biofeedback, reinforcement, or aversion therapy, to manage and improve the behavior of the client.

Care

The provision of accommodations, comfort, and care to an individual, implying responsibility for safety, including care, treatment, service, rehabilitation, habilitation, or other programs instituted by the organization for clients.

Care (or Treatment or Service) Plan

A plan, based on data gathered during individual assessment, that identifies the care needs of the client, lists the strategy for providing services to meet those needs, documents care goals and objectives, outlines the criteria for terminating specified interventions, and documents the progress of the client in meeting specified goals and objectives. The format of the plan in some organizations may be guided by individual-specific policies and procedures, protocols, practice guidelines, clinical paths, care maps, or a combination of several methods. The plan of care may include care, treatment, service, habilitation, and rehabilitation. *Care plan* is synonymous with the phrase *plan of care.*

Care Planning

Care planning addresses care, treatment, service, or program planning.

Case Management

The ongoing provision of service aimed at assessing needs of the clients, linking community resources, and delivering flexible problem solving and crisis response (such as assertive community treatment, wraparound services, and family preservation).

Case Manager

The individual primarily responsible for the care, treatment, or service of the client, or for seeing that necessary care is delivered. The phrase *case manager* is used interchangeably with *case coordinator, primary therapist, primary counselor, lead therapist,* and *lead counselor.*

Case Plan

Individualized planning and provision of services that address the needs, safety, and well-being of a child or youth while in foster care.

Child/Adolescent/Youth Behavioral Health Care

Behavioral health care services/programs for the assessment and/or care, treatment, or service of children, adolescents, or youths.

Child Psychiatrist, Qualified

A physician who specializes in assessing and treating children or adolescents with psychiatric disorders; who is fully licensed to practice medicine in the state in which he or she practices; and who has successfully completed an approved child psychiatry training program, has been certified in child psychiatry by the American Board of Psychiatry and Neurology, or has the documented equivalent in education, training, or experience.

Client

A person who receives care, treatment, or service. The term is synonymous with *patient, individual served, resident, consumer, youth, child,* and *recipient of treatment/care services.*

Clinical/Case Record

The account, compiled by health care professionals, of a variety of health information about the client, such as his or her psychiatric and medical history, present illness, findings on examination, details of care, and notes on progress.

Clinical/Case Record Administrator, Qualified

A registered record administrator who has successfully passed an appropriate examination conducted by the American Health Information Management Association, or who has the documented equivalent in education, training, or experience.

Clinical/Case Record Technician, Qualified

A record technician who has successfully passed the appropriate accreditation examination conducted by the American Health Information Management Association, or who has the documented equivalent in education, training, or experience.

Clinical Leader

A health care professional with overall responsibility to plan, organize, and operate a clinical service or program, such as the clinical director, discipline chief, unit or service director, clinical psychologist, social worker, psychiatric nurse, or qualified psychiatrist.

Clinical Privileges

Authorization granted by the appropriate authority (such as a governing body) to a practitioner to provide specific care services in an organization within well-defined limits, based on the following factors, as applicable: license, education, training, experience, competence, health status, and judgment.

Clinician

An individual charged with providing direct care, treatment, or service to clients.

Community

The individuals, families, groups, agencies, facilities, or institutions within the locality served by the health care organization.

Competency

The knowledge, skill, ability, and behavior that a person possesses in order to perform defined tasks correctly and skillfully.

Compliance

To act in accordance with stated requirements, such as standards. Levels of compliance include the following: does not provide evidence of acceptable compliance (most deficient); does not provide evidence of acceptable compliance (more deficient); does not provide evidence of acceptable compliance (least deficient); acceptable compliance; and good compliance.

Comprehensive Accreditation Manual for Behavioral Health Care (CAMBHC)

A single-volume publication consisting of policies and procedures relating to behavioral health care accreditation surveys and the delineation of current behavioral health care standards with the corresponding scoring guidelines, aggregation rules, and decision rules.

Concurrent Review

Evaluative activities conducted while the client is in active care.

Confidentiality

(1) Restriction of access to data and information to individuals who have a need, a reason, and permission for such access. (2) An individual's rights, within the law, to personal and informational privacy, including his or her health care records.

Consultation

Provision of professional advice or services on request.

Continuing Care

Care, treatment, or service provided over an extended time, in various settings, spanning the illness-to-wellness continuum.

Continuing Care Plan

A documented plan of action for a client developed before discharge or transfer to another level of care, treatment, or service. The purpose of the plan is to assist the client in sustaining the progress that has been achieved through linkage with supportive resources located in the environment to which the client is being returned. The continuing care plan is sometimes included within a discharge summary or is recorded in a separate planning document.

Continuity of Care
A component of care quality consisting of the degree to which the care, treatment, or service needed by a client is coordinated among practitioners, across organizations, and over time.

Continuum of Care
Matching the ongoing needs of the client with the appropriate level and type of medical, health, or psychosocial care, treatment, or service within an organization or across multiple organizations.

Coordination of Care
The process of coordinating care, treatment, or services provided by a health care organization, including referral to appropriate community resources and liaison with others (such as the individual's physician, other health care organizations, or community services involved in care), to meet the ongoing identified needs of the client, to ensure implementation of the plan of care, and to avoid unnecessary duplication of care, treatment, or services.

Corrections Services
Behavioral health care services provided in a correctional setting.

Credentialing
The process of obtaining, verifying, and assessing the qualifications of a health care practitioner to provide client care, treatment, or service in or for a health care organization.

Credentials
Documented evidence of licensure, education, training, experience, or other qualifications.

Crisis Stabilization
A highly structured environment for clients who require 24-hour registered nursing supervision and who may be incapable of self-preservation in case of an internal disaster. Crisis stabilization is typically characterized by a short length of stay with discharge or transfer to a hospital or community-treatment services.

Criteria
(1) Expected level(s) of achievement, or specifications against which performance or quality may be compared. (2) For purposes of eligibility for a Joint Commission survey, the conditions necessary for health care organizations and networks to be surveyed for accreditation by The Joint Commission.

Criteria for Discharge
Statements that guide staff in knowing when the client is ready for discharge or transfer. These criteria might be one and the same as clearly written objectives or can be separate statements included in the care plan. Discharge criteria should be consistent with or may be guided by any formal placement criteria such as Second Edition–Revised of its Patient Placement Criteria (ASAM PPC-2R) from the American Society of Addiction Medicine (ASAM) or Child and Adolescent Level of Care

Utilization System (CALOCUS) in development by the American Academy of Child and Adolescent Psychiatry and the American Association of Community Psychiatrists.

Critical Paths
See practice guidelines.

Cultural Assessment
An evaluation of the cultural influences on the existing value system of the client and how cultural/ethnic influences affect the conditions that bring him or her to care, treatment, or service. Cultural influences include ethnicity, race, gender, geography, and socioeconomic status.

Data
Uninterpreted material, facts, or clinical observations.

Department
Any structural unit of the behavioral health care organization, whether it is called a department, service, unit, or something similar.

Detoxification
The systematic reduction of the amount of a toxic agent in the body or the elimination of a toxic agent from the body.

Diagnosis
A scientifically or medically acceptable term given to a complex of symptoms (disturbances of function or sensation of which the client is aware), signs (disturbances the physician or another client can detect), and findings (detected by laboratory, x-ray, or other diagnostic procedures, or responses to therapy).

Diagnostic Testing
Laboratory and other invasive, diagnostic, and imaging procedures.

Dimensions of Performance
Nine definable, measurable, and improvable attributes of organization performance related to "doing the right things right" (appropriateness, availability, and efficacy) and "doing things well" (timeliness, effectiveness, continuity, safety, efficiency, and respect and caring).

Director
A person who directs, controls, supervises, or manages an organization or a component thereof.

Discharge
The point at which the involvement of the client with an organization/program is terminated and the organization/program no longer maintains active responsibility for the care of the client.

Discharge Planning
A formalized process in a health care organization through which a program of continuing and

follow-up care, treatment, or service is planned and carried out for each client. Discharge planning encompasses a documented sequence of tasks and activities designed to achieve, within projected time frames, stated goals that lead to the timely release of clients to either their homes or to facilities or programs with a lower level of care, treatment, or service. Discharge planning is undertaken to ensure that clients remain in a health care organization only for as long as needed.

Documentation
The process of recording information in the clinical/case record and other source documents.

Drug
Any substance, other than food or devices, that may be used on or administered to persons as an aid in the diagnosis, care, treatment, or prevention of disease or other abnormal conditions. Synonymous with *medication.*

Drug Administration
The act of giving a prescribed and prepared dose of an identified drug to the client.

Drug Allergies
A state of hypersensitivity induced by exposure to a particular drug antigen resulting in harmful immunologic reactions on subsequent drug exposures, such as a penicillin drug allergy.

Drug Dispensing
The issuance of one or more doses of a prescribed medication by a pharmacist or other authorized staff member to another person responsible for administering it.

Drug History
A drug history includes, but is not limited to, the following: drugs used in the past; drugs used recently, particularly within the preceding 48 hours; drugs of preference; frequency with which each drug is used; route of administration of each drug; drugs used in combination; dosages used; year of first use of each drug; previous occurrences of overdose, withdrawal, or adverse drug reactions; and history of previous treatment for alcohol or drug abuse.

Effectiveness
The degree to which the care is provided in the correct manner, given the current state of knowledge, to achieve the desired or projected outcome(s) for the client.

Efficacy
The degree to which the care, treatment, or service of the client has been shown to accomplish the desired or projected outcome(s).

Efficiency
The relationship between the outcomes (results of care) and the resources used to deliver care.

Electroconvulsive Therapy
A form of somatic treatment using electricity to evoke a convulsive response.

Emergency

(1) An unexpected or sudden occasion, such as emergency surgery needed to prevent death or serious disability. (2) A natural or man-made event that significantly disrupts the environment of care (for example, damage to the organization's building[s] and grounds due to severe winds, storms, or earthquakes); that significantly disrupts care, treatment, and service (for example, loss of utilities, such as power, water, or telephones, due to floods, civil disturbances, accidents, or emergencies in the organization or its community); or that results in sudden, significantly changed or increased demands for the organization's services (for example, bioterrorist attack, building collapse, or plane crash in the organization's community). Some emergencies are called disasters or potential injury creating events (PICEs).

Emergency-management Plan

A component of an organization's environment of care program designed to manage the consequences of natural disasters or other emergencies that disrupt the organization's ability to provide care, treatment, and service. *See also* emergency.

Emotional and Behavioral Assessment

The evaluation of the emotional, behavioral, and cognitive functioning of the client, conducted by a variety of professionals who have been deemed competent to conduct such assessments by virtue of licensure and/or organizational standards. It is conducted at the time of intake and continuously thereafter during care, treatment, or service. It includes an evaluation of current emotional and behavioral functioning, history of emotional and behavioral problems and/or treatment, family history of psychological problems, cognitive functioning, maladaptive or problem behaviors, history of addictive behaviors by individuals or by family members, addictive behaviors such as drug abuse or gambling, and emotional and behavioral functioning.

Entry

The process by which the client is screened and/or assessed by the organization or the practitioner in order to determine the capabilities of the organization or practitioner to provide the care, treatment, or service required to meet the needs of the client.

Equipment Maintenance, Preventive

The planned, scheduled, visual, mechanical, engineering, and functional evaluation of equipment conducted before using new equipment and at specified intervals throughout the equipment's lifetime. The purpose is to maintain equipment performance within manufacturers' guidelines and specifications and to help ensure accurate diagnosis, treatment, or monitoring. It includes measuring performance specifications and evaluating specific safety factors.

Equipment Maintenance, Routine

The performance of basic safety checks—that is, the visual, technical, and functional evaluations of equipment—to identify obvious deficiencies before they have a negative impact. It normally includes inspections of the case, power cord, structural frame, enclosure, controls, indicators, and so on, as appropriate.

Error

An unintended act, either of omission or commission, or an act that does not achieve its intended outcome.

Family

The person(s) who plays a significant role in the individual's life. This may include an individual(s) not legally related to the client. This person(s) is often referred to as a surrogate decision maker if authorized to make care decisions for a client, should the individual lose decision-making capacity. *See also* guardian; surrogate decision maker.

Family Preservation

Organizations providing and/or coordinating services for a child/adolescent and his or her family with the goal of maintaining the child/adolescent in her or his family and/or community.

Forensic Program or Services

Behavioral health care services provided by an order issued by the criminal or juvenile justice system.

Foster Care, Traditional

A living arrangement in which a child/adolescent resides outside his or her own home in a single residence as a means of providing protection and shelter. These living arrangements are private, single residences, which include relative and nonrelative foster homes and nonfinalized adoptive homes.

Function

(1) A goal-directed, interrelated series of processes, such as individual assessment or individual care. (2) A quality, trait, or fact that is so related to another as to be dependent on and to vary with this other, as when the success of the endeavor is a function of the commitment of management and employees to continuously improving performance and the quality of services.

Functional Assessment

Assessing the functional status of the client; the ability to perform age-appropriate tasks of self-care and self-fulfillment. Functional status may be broken down into physical functions (for example, independent in self-care) and psychosocial functions (such as the ability to participate in education or work, engage in leisure activities, and have adequate social relationships).

Goals

Broad and encompassing statements of desirable behavioral change that a client should achieve to reflect a maximum or optimal care outcome. (Some providers use the term *long-term goals* or *long-term objectives*.) A logical and specific relationship should exist between each goal and each identified active problem/need. *See also* problems/needs list.

Guardian

A parent, trustee, conservator, committee, or other individual or agency empowered by law to act on behalf of, or be responsible for, an individual. *See also* family; surrogate decision maker.

Improve

To take actions that result in the desired measurable change.

Incident Report

Documentation of an event that varies from established policies and procedures pertaining to care, treatment, or service.

Indicator

A measure to determine, over time, an organization's performance of functions, processes, and outcomes.

Infection Control Program (or Process)

An organizationwide program, including policies and procedures, for the surveillance, prevention, and control of infection.

Information

Interpreted sets of data that can assist in decision-making.

In-home Behavioral Health Care Services

Behavioral health care, treatment, or service provided in the residence of a client. In-home behavioral health care services may include individual and family counseling, mobile crisis evaluation services, or early intervention services.

Inpatient Program

A program, in a suitably equipped setting not eligible for survey as a hospital program under the *Comprehensive Accreditation Manual for Hospitals (CAMH),* that provides services to persons who require care that warrants 24-hour treatment or habilitation.

Inpatient Services

A highly structured environment for individuals who require 24-hour registered nursing supervision and who may be incapable of self-preservation in case of an internal disaster.

In-service

Organized education designed to enhance the skills of organization staff members or teach them new skills relevant to their responsibilities and disciplines.

Interventions

Planned procedures designed by the staff to bring about the behavioral changes identified in the care objectives. Interventions include any assignments given to the client. The frequency of interventions and the name of the provider (whenever possible) or the discipline responsible for carrying out the intervention should be documented. Interventions may also be identified as strategies, methods, steps, or modalities.

Knowledge-based Information

A collection of stored facts, models, and information that can be used for designing and redesigning processes and for problem solving. In the context of this manual, knowledge-based information is found in clinical, scientific, and management literature.

Laboratory

See Pathology and Clinical Laboratory Services.

Licensed Independent Practitioner

Any individual permitted by law and by the organization to provide care, treatment, and services to the client without direction or supervision, within the scope of the individual's licensure or certification, and in accordance with individually granted clinical responsibilities (these individuals may be referred to by other terms such as *independent care provider*). In many behavioral health care organizations, licensed independent practitioners include physicians, psychologists, and social workers.

Licensed Practical Nurse

A nurse who has completed a practical nursing program and is licensed by a state to provide routine care of clients under the direction of a registered nurse or a physician. Referred to as licensed vocational nurse (LVN) in California and Texas.

Licensure

A legal right that is granted by a government agency in compliance with a statute governing an occupation (such as medicine or nursing) or the operation of an activity (such as in a behavioral health care organization).

Life Domains

Spheres of life concerns or functions, which may include health, nutrition, environment, spirituality, military, financial, social, sexual, family, leisure, peer relationships, vocational, educational, legal, cultural, emotional, behavioral, addictions, and cognition.

Long-term Goals or Objectives

See Goals.

Measure

To collect quantifiable data about a function or process.

Measurement

The systematic process of data collection, repeated over time or at a single point in time.

Medical Facility

As defined by the American Hospital Association, an organization classified as providing individual care services in buildings designed for both overnight and day-only or night-only services, including, for example, residential treatment facilities, ambulatory clinics, hospitals, and long term care facilities.

Medical History

A component of the clinical/case record consisting of an account of the history of the client, obtained whenever possible from the individual, and including at least the following information: chief complaint, details of the present illness or care needs, relevant history, and relevant inventory by body system.

Medical Laboratory Services

Clinical laboratory tests conducted for the client, either directly by the health care organization or as a contracted service, for the purpose of obtaining specific information about the condition of the individual.

Medication

Any substance, other than food or devices, that may be used on or administered to persons as an aid in the diagnosis, care, treatment, or prevention of disease or other abnormal conditions. Synonymous with *drug.*

Medication Error

A discrepancy between what a physician orders and what is reported to have occurred. Types of medication errors include omission, unauthorized drug, extra dose, wrong dose, wrong dosage form, wrong rate, deteriorated drug, wrong administration technique, and wrong time.

An omission medication error is the failure to give an ordered dose; a refused dose is not counted as an error if the nurse responsible for administering the dose tried, but failed, to persuade the patient to take it. Doses withheld according to written policies, such as for x-ray procedures, are not counted as omission errors. An unauthorized drug medication error is the administration of a dose of medication not authorized to be given to that client. Instances of brand or therapeutic substitution are counted as unauthorized medication errors only when prohibited by organization policy. A wrong dose medication error occurs when a client receives an amount of medicine that is greater than or less than the amount ordered; the range of allowable deviation is based on each organization's definition. *See also* sentinel event; significant medication errors, and significant adverse drug reactions.

Mental Retardation Professional, Qualified

A person who has been determined by the organization, based on the person's education, training, or experience, to have the ability to obtain and interpret information about a person with developmental disabilities in terms of the needs of the client and an understanding of the range, intensity, and duration of care, treatment, service, or habilitation needed in the care of the client.

Mission Statement

A written expression that sets forth the purpose of an organization or one of its components. The generation of a mission statement usually precedes the formation of goals and objectives of the organization.

Multidisciplinary Team

A group of providers composed of representatives of a range of professions, disciplines, or service areas.

Needs

See Problems; Problems/Needs List.

Normalization

The act or process of making available, to developmentally disabled clients, patterns and conditions of everyday life that are as similar as possible to those of the mainstream of society. This allows clients to enjoy a manner of living close to that considered normal in the community. The basic principle is that what is offered represents the least departure from normal patterns of living that can be effective in meeting the developmental needs of clients.

Nurse, Qualified, Psychiatric

A licensed, registered nurse who has a master's degree in psychiatric nursing, who has been certified to practice psychiatric nursing by the voluntary certification process of the American Nurses' Association, or who has the documented equivalent in education, training, or experience.

Nursing Care

Professional processes intended to assist a client in the performance of those activities contributing to health or recovery that he or she would perform unaided if he or she had the necessary strength, will, or knowledge. This includes, but is not limited to, assisting clients in carrying out therapeutic plans and understanding their health needs. The special content of nursing care varies in different countries and situations, and, as defined, it is not given solely by registered nurses, but also by other health care professionals.

Nursing Staff

Registered nurses, licensed practical or vocational nurses, nursing assistants, and other nursing personnel who perform nursing care in a health care organization.

Nutrients

Proteins, carbohydrates, lipids, vitamins, electrolytes, minerals, and water.

Nutrition

The sum of the processes by which one takes in and uses nutrients.

Nutrition Assessment

A comprehensive approach to defining the nutritional status of the client that combines medical, nutrition, and medication intake histories; physical examinations; anthropometric measurements; and laboratory data.

Nutrition Care

Interventions and counseling of clients regarding appropriate nutrition intake by integrating information from the nutrition assessment with information on food and other sources of nutrients and meal preparation consistent with cultural background and socioeconomic status. Nutrition therapy, a component of medical treatment, includes eternal and parenteral nutrition.

Nutrition Screening

The process of identifying characteristics known to be associated with nutrition problems in order to determine if clients are malnourished or at a high risk for malnourishment. Screening facilitates effective intervention.

Objectives

Statements of desirable, observable, and, where possible, measurable behavioral change that demonstrate the achievement of the steps necessary to meet the goal. For instance, in problem-oriented care plans, the objectives reflect the measurable behavioral changes that demonstrate the elimination or significant reduction of the identified individual problems. In need-oriented care plans, the objectives reflect the measurable behavioral changes that demonstrate the gaining of knowledge or insight, the planning, practicing/gaining skills or application of skills to particular situations. Objectives are directly related to the goals and the identified active problems/needs. The phrase *short-term goals* is sometimes used instead of *objectives*. In rare instances, other terms, such as *challenges*, are used. Each objective should include an anticipated time frame of achievement.

Occupational Therapist, Qualified, Certified

An individual who is a graduate of an occupational therapy program accredited by a nationally recognized accrediting body; is currently certified as an occupational therapist by the American Occupational Therapy Certification Board; meets any current legal requirements of licensure or registration; or has the documented equivalence in education, training, and experience and is currently competent in the field. The qualified occupational therapist uses purposeful, goal-oriented activities in assessing, evaluating, and/or treating persons whose function is impaired by physical illness or injury, emotional disorder, congenital or developmental disability, or the aging process, to achieve optimum functioning, to prevent disability, and to maintain health.

Organizationwide

Throughout the organization and across multiple structural and staffing components, as appropriate.

Orientation

A process to provide initial training and information and to assess staff members' competence related to their job responsibilities and the mission, vision, and values of the organization.

Outcome

The result of the performance (or nonperformance) of a function or process(es).

Outpatient Program

Behavioral health care organizations providing care, treatment, or service on an appointment system for each visit.

Partial-Hospitalization/Day Treament/Adult Day Care/ Intensive Outpatient Services

An environment offering an organized day or night program of assessment, care, treatment, service, habilitation, or rehabilitation for clients not requiring 24-hour care. For behavioral health care, this may be a structured, ongoing program that typically meets two to five times a week, for two to five hours per day.

Pathology and Clinical Laboratory Services

The services that provide information on diagnosis, prevention, or treatment of disease through the examination of the structural and functional changes in tissues and organs of the body that cause or are caused by disease.

Performance

The way in which an individual, group, or organization carries out or accomplishes its important functions and processes.

Performance Improvement

The continuous study and adaptation of functions and processes of a health care organization to increase the probability of achieving desired outcomes and to better meet the needs of the individuals and other users of services. This is the third segment of a performance measurement, assessment, and improvement system.

Performance Measure

A quantitative tool (for example, rate, ratio, index, or percentage) that provides an indication of an organization's performance in relation to a specified process or outcome.

Personnel Record

The complete employment record of a staff member or an employee, including job application, education and employment history, job description, performance evaluation(s), and, when applicable, evidence of current licensure, certification, or registration.

Pharmaceutical Equivalence

The degree to which two formulations of the same medication are identical in strength, concentration, and dosage form.

Pharmacist

An individual who has a degree in pharmacy and is licensed and registered to prepare, preserve, compound, and dispense drugs and chemicals.

Physical Assessment in 24-Hour Settings

Physicians and nursing personnel (or a community source) may conduct the evaluation of the physical needs of the client. It includes a medical history and physical exam. (*Note*: The physical assessment will also include review and evaluation of any applicable lab work requested as part of the physical exam.)

For children, youth, and persons with developmental disabilities, the physical assessment should also include an evaluation of motor development and functioning; sensorimotor functioning; speech, hearing, and language functioning; oral health and oral hygiene; visual functioning; and immunization status.

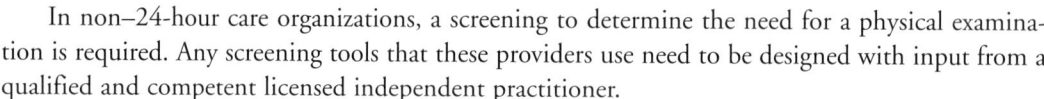

In non–24-hour care organizations, a screening to determine the need for a physical examination is required. Any screening tools that these providers use need to be designed with input from a qualified and competent licensed independent practitioner.

Physical Therapist, Qualified

An individual who is a graduate of a physical therapist education program accredited by a nationally recognized accreditation body; meets any current legal requirements of licensure or registration; or has the documented equivalence in training, education, or experience; and is currently competent in the field.

Physician, Qualified

A doctor of medicine or doctor of osteopathy who, by virtue of education, training, and demonstrated competence, is granted clinical responsibilities (or "privileges") by the organization to perform specific diagnostic or therapeutic procedure(s) and who is fully licensed to practice medicine.

Plan

To formulate or describe the approach to achieving the goals related to improving the performance of the organization.

Plan of Care

A plan, based on data gathered during individual assessment, that identifies the care needs of the client, lists the strategy for providing services to meet those needs, documents care goals and objectives, outlines the criteria for terminating specified interventions, and documents the progress of the client in meeting specified goals and objectives. The format of the plan in some organizations may be guided by individual-specific policies and procedures, protocols, practice guidelines, clinical paths, care maps, or a combination of several methods. The plan of care may include care, treatment, service, habilitation, and rehabilitation. This phrase is synonymous with *care plan*.

Policies and Procedures

The act, method, or manner of proceeding in some process, or course of action; a particular course of action or way of doing something.

Practice Guidelines

Descriptive tools or standardized specifications for care of the typical client in the typical situation, developed through a formal process that incorporates the best scientific evidence of effectiveness with expert opinion. Synonyms or near synonyms include *clinical criteria, critical paths, parameter* (or *practice parameter*), *protocol, algorithm, review criteria, preferred practice pattern,* and *guidelines.*

Preparedness Activities

Those activities an organization undertakes to build capacity and identify resources that may be used if an emergency occurs.

Prescribing or Ordering

Directing the selection, preparation, or administration of medication(s).

Problems

Demonstrable, observable behaviors that create difficulty for the client or interfere with the ability to carry out the skills of daily living or result in dysfunction.

Problems/Needs List

A formal, written problems or needs list is not required by The Joint Commission. However, as a result of the completion of the data collection and assessment, the provider should be aware of all the problems or deficits of the client. These will be sorted into three groups: problems for which care, treatment, or service will be provided; problems to be deferred; and problems for which referral is indicated. These three groups constitute the problems/needs list. This may be a written list or merely the conceptualization of the prioritized care needs of the client. This is the process that leads to the "clinical or case formulation." Again, these may be written or demonstrated through a comprehensive care plan. The end result is prioritization of care, either through a comprehensive care plan, a case conference, or other process.

Procedure

(1) A series of steps taken to accomplish a desired end, as in a therapeutic, cosmetic, or surgical procedure. (2) A unit of health care, as in services and procedures.

Process

A goal-directed, interrelated series of actions, events, mechanisms, or steps.

Program

An outline of work to be done or a prearranged plan or procedure, as in "the administration's program." A general term for an organized system of services designed to address the treatment/care needs of the individual being served.

Progress Notes

Sequential narratives that depict the progress of the client in relation to the care plan. They may also be used to record other significant events.

Protective Services

A range of sociolegal, assistive, and remedial services that facilitate the exercise of individual rights and provide certain supportive and surrogate mechanisms. Such mechanisms are designed to assist developmentally disabled clients to obtain the maximum independence possible while protecting them from exploitation, neglect, or abuse. Depending on the nature and extent of individual needs, protective services may range from counseling to full guardianship.

Provider

Staff providing direct care, treatment, or service to clients, not to organizations.

Psychiatric Nurse, Qualified

See Nurse, Qualified, Psychiatric.

Psychiatrist, Qualified

A physician who specializes in the assessment and treatment of persons having psychiatric disorders, is certified by the American Board of Psychiatry and Neurology, or has the documented equivalent in education, training, or experience, and is fully licensed to practice medicine in the state in which he or she practices.

Psychodrama Therapy

The use of action methods of enactment, sociometry, group dynamics, role theory, and social systems analysis to facilitate constructive change in individuals and groups by developing new perceptions or reorganizing old cognitive patterns and concomitant changes in behavior.

Psychologist, Qualified

A person who either possesses a doctoral degree in psychology or has the documented equivalent in education, training, or experience, and who meets current legal requirements of licensure, registration, or certification in the state in which he or she renders services. An individual who specializes and is licensed in psychological research, testing, or therapy.

Psychosocial Assessment

The evaluation of psychological and social functioning of the client, including conflicts or problems involving environment and living situation; leisure and recreation; religious and spiritual orientation; childhood history; military service history; financial issues; usual social, peer-group, and environmental setting; sexual history; family circumstances; mental status (when indicated); psychiatric evaluation (when indicated); psychological evaluation (when indicated); and history of previous behavioral problems and/or care, treatment, or service.

The evaluation also includes determining the appropriateness and level of need for the inclusion of the family of the client. It also includes a clinical analysis of these data in consideration of care needs. Age or clinical considerations may determine data needs. Family circumstances include the constellation of the family group; current living situation; and social, ethnic, cultural, emotional, and health factors.

Qualified Individual

An individual or staff member who is qualified to participate in one or all of the mechanisms outlined in the standards by virtue of the following: education, training, experience, competence, registration, certification, or applicable licensure, law or regulation.

Quality Control

The performance of processes through which actual performance is measured and compared with goals, and the difference is acted on.

Quality Improvement

An approach to the continuous study and improvement of the processes of providing health care services to meet the needs of individuals and others. Synonyms include *continuous quality improvement, continuous improvement, organizationwide performance improvement,* and *total quality management.*

Reassessment

Ongoing data collection that begins on initial assessment, comparing the most recent data with the data collected on the previous assessment.

Recreational Therapist, Qualified

An individual who, at a minimum, is a graduate of a baccalaureate degree program in recreational therapy accredited by a nationally recognized accreditation body; is currently a Certified Therapeutic Recreation Specialist (CTRS) by the National Council for Therapeutic Recreation Certification (NCTRC); meets any current legal requirements of licensure, registration, or certification; or has the documented equivalence in education, training, or experience; and is currently competent in the field.

Reference Database

An organized collection of similar data from many organizations that can be used to compare an organization's performance to that of others.

Referral

The sending of a client, either for consultation or for care, treatment, or service (1) from one clinician to another clinician or specialist, (2) from one setting or service to another, or (3) from one physician (the referring physician) to another physician (or some other resource).

Registered Nurse

An individual who is qualified by an approved postsecondary program or baccalaureate or higher degree in nursing and licensed by the state, commonwealth, or territory to practice professional nursing.

Religious/Spiritual Assessment

Part of the psychosocial assessment. The spiritual assessment evaluates such factors as the philosophical orientation of the client toward the purpose and meaning of life, relationship with humanity (degree of isolation, degree of alienation from others), and with God or a higher power. It is not solely intended to identify the religion or religious practices of the client, but also to analyze how (if at all) the spiritual orientation of the client affects his or her lifestyle.

Residential Program

A program that provides 24-hour care, treatment, and services to clients who need a less structured environment than that of an inpatient program and who are capable of self-preservation in the event of an internal disaster. A residential setting may serve children, adolescents, or adults.

Respect and Caring

The degree to which those providing services do so with sensitivity for the needs, expectations, and individual differences of the client. This also includes the degree to which the client or a designee is involved in his or her own care decisions.

Retrospective Review

Evaluative activities conducted when the client is no longer in active treatment.

Risk-Management Activities

Clinical and administrative activities that organizations undertake to identify, evaluate, and reduce the risk of injury to clients, personnel, and visitors and the risk of loss to the organization itself.

Safety

The degree to which the risk of an intervention (for example, use of a drug or a procedure) and risk in the care environment are reduced for the client and others, including the behavioral health care provider.

Safety Management

A component of an organization's management of the environment of care program that maintains and improves the general safety of the care environment of the client.

Scope of Care and Services

The activities performed by governance, managerial, clinical, or support personnel.

Screening

The process of evaluating the physical functioning and psychosocial (a combination of psychological and social evaluations) functioning of the client to determine the need for further assessment or care, treatment, or service. Screening also begins the process of determining appropriate care, treatment, or service for the client.

Sentinel Event

An unexpected occurrence involving death or serious physical or psychological injury, or risk thereof. *Serious injury* specifically includes loss of limb or function. The phrase "or risk thereof" includes any process variation for which a recurrence would carry a significant chance of a serious adverse outcome. *See also* Medication Error; Significant Medication Errors and Significant Adverse Drug Reactions.

Service(s)

Structural divisions of an organization or its staff; also the delivery of care, treatment, or service.

Side Effect

A result of a drug or other therapy in addition to, or in extension of, the desired therapeutic effect.

Significant Medication Errors and Significant Adverse Drug Reactions

Unintended, undesirable, and unexpected effects of prescribed medications or of medication errors that require discontinuing a medication or modifying the dose, require initial or prolonged hospitalization, result in disability, require treatment with a prescription medication, result in cognitive deterioration or impairment, are life threatening, result in death, or result in congenital anomalies. *See also* Medication Error; Sentinel Event.

Social Worker, Qualified

An individual who either has met the requirements of a graduate curriculum (leading to a master's degree) in a school of social work that is accredited by the Council on Social Work Education or who has the documented equivalent in education, training, or experience. For purposes of Joint Commission Medicare surveys, social workers meet the personnel requirements outlined in the Medicare regulations for home care agencies.

Speech-Language Pathologist, Qualified

An individual who holds either a master's or doctoral degree; the Certificate of Clinical Competence (CCC) of the American Speech-Language–Hearing Association (ASHA); and where applicable, state licensure; or has the documented equivalent education, training, or experience.

Speech Screening

A process that may include such tests as articulation in connected speech and formal testing situations; voice, in terms of judgments of pitch, intensity, and quality and in terms of determinations of appropriate vocal hygiene; and fluency, usually measured in terms of frequency and severity of stuttering or dysfluency (based on evaluation of speech flow-sequence, duration, rhythm, rate, and fluency).

Spiritual/Religious Assessment

See Religious/Spiritual Assessment.

Staff

Individuals, such as employees, volunteers, contractors, or temporary agency personnel, who provide services in the organization. *See also* licensed independent practitioner.

Staff, Medical, or Licensed Independent Practitioner

Individuals who successfully complete a credentialing process and are granted clinical privileges by the organization.

Staffing Effectiveness

The number, competence, and skill mix of staff as related to the provision of needed services.

Standard

A statement that defines the performance expectations, structures, or processes that must be substantially in place in an organization to enhance the quality of care, treatment, or service.

Surrogate Decision Maker

Someone appointed to act on behalf of another. Surrogates make decisions only when a client is without capacity or has given permission to involve others. *See also* Advocate; Family.

Systematic

Pursuing a defined objective(s) in a planned, step-by-step manner.

Therapeutic Equivalence

The degree to which two formulations of different active ingredients are judged by the clinical staff to have acceptably similar therapeutic effects.

Therapeutic Foster Care

For the purposes of Joint Commission accreditation, intensive services provided to no more than two clients in treatment in a single residence. Services are delivered primarily by treatment foster parents who bear direct responsibility for implementing the select in-home aspects of the care plan.

Timeliness

The degree to which the care is provided to the client at the most beneficial or necessary time.

Transfer

The formal shifting of responsibility for the care of a client (1) from one care unit to another, (2) from one clinical service to another, (3) from the care of one licensed independent practitioner to another, or (4) from one organization to another organization.

Transitional Living/Supervised Care/Supportive Living

A 24-hour living arrangement provided to clients in need of a supportive environment. This level of care is typically provided as a community reentry phase within a care continuum and may serve adults or older adolescents.

Treatment/Care Plan

See Care Plan; Plan of Care.

Utilization Management

The examination and evaluation of the appropriateness of the utilization of an organization's resources. Also referred to as a utilization review.

Variance

(1) A measure of the differences in a set of observations. (2) In statistics, equal to the square of the standard deviation.

Variation

The differences in results obtained in measuring the same phenomenon more than once. The sources of variation in a process over time can be grouped into two major classes: common causes and special causes.

Vocational Rehabilitation

A service or program designed to attain, retain, or restore vocational usefulness of persons experiencing limited functioning. Vocational rehabilitation services may include vocational evaluation services, employment skills training, work activities, and supportive employment.

Waived Tests

Tests that meet the Clinical Laboratory Improvement Amendments of 1988 requirements for waived tests; they are cleared by the Food and Drug Administration (FDA) for home use and employ methodologies that are so simple and accurate as to render the likelihood of erroneous results negligible or pose no risk or harm to the individual tested if the test is performed incorrectly. Examples include dipstick urinalysis, glucometers, and urine pregnancy testing. A certificate of waiver needs to be obtained from the Centers for Medicare & Medicaid Services (CMS, formerly known as HCFA) and be available for review by the surveyor(s).

Wraparound Services

See Family Preservation.

Index